NU

MW01204156

The Manning Company

Skidmore-Roth Publishing

Developmental Editor: TOM LOCHHAAS

Printed in the United States of America

The Manning Company
11756 Borman Drive, Suite 202
St. Louis, Missouri 63146-4133

Skidmore-Roth Publishing
207 Cincinnati Avenue
El Paso, Texas 79902-9945

ISBN 0-944132-15-4

NURSE ASSISTANT HANDBOOK

EDITORIAL BOARD

Manning Skidmore Roth
St. Louis • El Paso • 1990

CONTENTS

iii

vi

Chapter 1
Functions of the Nurse Assistant

This chapter includes information on the following:
Roles and responsibilities
Personal characteristics
Personal hygiene and appearance
Ethical and legal behavior
Principles for interacting with patients

Roles and Responsibilities

▸ Your specific roles and responsibilities depend on facility policy.
▸ Generally you are an assistant to the nurse, who supervises your work.
▸ You should perform only tasks for which you have been specifically trained.
▸ Responsibilities in patient care:
  • Assist in admitting the patient
  • Assist patients with personal hygiene
  • Assist patients with positioning, moving, and being transported
  • Assist in serving meals and feeding patients
  • Measure patients' fluid intake and output
  • Assist patients with elimination functions
  • Assist with specimen collection
  • Perform procedures for the patient with an elimination problem
  • Perform heat and cold applications
  • Assist patients with range of motion exercises

- Assist in patient rehabilitation procedures
- Take patients' vital signs
- Use patient safety devices as directed
- Provide care in emergencies until help arrives
- Maintain control against infection
- Assist with care for the orthopedic patient
- Assist with care for the surgical patient
- Assist with care for the elderly patient
- Provide care for patients with common medical conditions
- Carry out special procedures as ordered
- Provide care for the dying patient
- Provide patient care in the home, if so trained
- Perform other tasks as directed by the nurse
► Responsibilities in the unit:
- Make beds
- Clean unit as directed
- Clean equipment as directed
- Maintain safety measures and patient protection
- Follow all facility policies for uniform wear and personal standards

Personal Characteristics

► Be trustworthy and dependable to the patient and other facility staff.
► Be sensitive to the patient's needs and considerate of the patient's feelings; look at things from the patient's point of view.
► Show respect and courtesy to the patient, family and visitors, and other facility staff. Help maintain the patient's and family's dignity by

calling them by name. Terms like "honey" or "dear" may be insulting.

- Be honest at all times.
- Be conscientious in carrying out all duties and activities.
- Maintain a cheerful attitude in your work; keep your emotions under control.
- Have patience in your interaction with co-workers and patients.

Personal Hygiene and Appearance

- Always follow your facility's dress code. Keep uniform clean and pressed. Wear clean clothes every day.
- Do not wear jewelry except a wedding or engagement ring if allowed. Wear a wristwatch with a second hand.
- Keep your hair brushed and in place, off your collar and not falling in your face.
- Use only minimal makeup and scents.
- Keep nails clean and short, using only clear polish.
- Wear comfortable shoes with good support. Polish them frequently and maintain a neat appearance.
- Exercise regularly.
- Follow a nutritious diet.
- If you smoke, try joining a smoking cessation program. Never smoke near patients and always wash hands immediately afterwards.
- Get sufficient rest so that you are always alert at work.

► Maintain good personal hygiene:
  • Bathe daily; use antiperspirant or deodorant.
  • Brush and floss teeth regularly; use mouthwash.
  • Prevent foot odor.

Ethical and Legal Behavior

► Always follow established ethical principles in your interactions with patients, staff, and all others:
  • Take no action you have not been trained to do or that is not in your responsibilities as a nurse assistant.
  • Respect all patients as individuals and accept their right to different beliefs.
  • Perform all duties ordered as faithfully and conscientiously as you can; report to the nurse any difficulties or problems you experience in carrying out your duties.
  • Help your patients as fully and sincerely as you can, never limiting yourself to only what the job requires.
► Always be aware of your legal responsibilities:
  • Keep all information about patients confidential; otherwise, you violate the patient's legal right to privacy.
  • Always perform actions following the accepted standards of care, and do not neglect to perform the correct actions in patient care; otherwise, you may be guilty of negligence.
  • You are responsible for your own actions, even when following orders; otherwise, if you perform an action you are not trained or

legally allowed to do, you may be guilty of negligence even if you were ordered to do it.

- Do not gossip or talk about patients, co-workers, or anyone else; otherwise, any negative implication of what you say may make you guilty of defamation of character.
- Do not provide care against the patient's wishes or perform actions you have not explained first to the patient; otherwise, you are violating the patient's right to give informed consent before care.
- Never discriminate against any person in any way because of the person's race, sex, religion, ethnic background, age, or any handicap; otherwise, you are violating the person's civil rights.
- Never leave the patient at a time of need without ensuring that a replacement provides care; otherwise, you are guilty of abandonment.
- Follow facility policy for reporting any accident or incident that is not part of routine care; otherwise, you may be guilty of negligence.
- Never touch the patient's body or threaten to touch the body without consent; otherwise, you may be guilty of battery or assault.
- Do not unnecessarily restrain or prevent free movement of a patient; otherwise, you may be guilty of false imprisonment.
- Good Samaritan laws protect you when you act to give care in an emergency, as long as you act within your training and to the best of your ability.

Principles for Interacting with Patients

- Act within the roles and responsibilities listed above.
- Demonstrate the good personal characteristics listed above.
- Act ethically and legally as described above.
- Be punctual in reporting to work and in carrying out scheduled patient duties.
- Help the patient willingly whenever asked.
- Listen to patients' complaints and problems and do what you can to help; report problems to the nurse.
- Do not talk to the patient about your own problems.
- Help the patient maintain confidence in the facility and other staff; never say anything negative about anyone else in the facility.
- If the patient is angry or hostile, do not take it personally, because many other factors can result in strong emotions. Always keep control over your own emotions. If your feelings become difficult to control, leave the patient in a safe situation and share your feelings with the nurse; get the support you need to continue with effective patient care.
- Praise and encourage patients as they improve or cope with a condition.
- Be aware that the patient's body language and expressions may reveal something the patient's words do not; for example, some patients may not want to admit they feel pain or are confused.

- ► Never talk to an elderly or ill patient like a child; patients can be easily offended by what may seem a condescending attitude.
- ► Interact courteously with the patient's family or other visitors following the same guidelines as for the patient.

Chapter 2
Safety

This chapter includes information on the following:
Principles of safety in the health care facility
General rules for fire safety
General rules for electrical safety
General rules for using restraints
Procedure: Applying a safety belt
Procedure: Applying a jacket restraint
Procedure: Applying mitt restraints
Procedure: Applying elbow restraints
Procedure: Applying ankle and wrist restraints

Principles of Safety in the Health Care Facility

- Infants and small children should never be left alone; keep plastic sheeting and bags away from children.
- The side rails of cribs should always be up and locked in place.
- Always assist elderly patients who may be in danger of falling.
- Always check the patient's identification bracelet and call the patient's name before performing any procedure.
- Give special assistance to any patients with impaired vision or hearing.
- Pay special attention to patients at risk of falling or other injury because of the side effects of their medication.
- To prevent choking, be sure the patient takes small bites of food and chews slowly.

- Keep the bed side rails up for unconscious or disoriented patients or when ordered for any patient.
- Except when providing care, keep the bed in the lowest possible position. Keep the wheels locked.
- Be sure the patient's signal light is always within reach. Always answer a patient's call promptly.
- Be sure the patient's slippers have nonskid soles.
- When transporting a patient by wheelchair or stretcher, take care the patient's feet stay in position to avoid injury. Be especially careful going around corners.
- Any time you cannot read a handwritten instruction or do not understand a written order or a label on a container or equipment, ask the nurse before proceeding with the procedure.
- Any time you see a potential hazard, such as a lighting problem or loose carpeting or floor tiles, report it immediately.
- Help the patient maintain good body alignment when positioned in bed or a wheelchair.
- Prevent the patient from being burned by hot food or hot bathing water.
- Clean up any spills on the floor immediately.
- Encourage the patient to use hand rails in the bathroom and elsewhere.
- Prevent the patient from being burned by hot food, hot bath water, hot soaks, or heating pads.

General Rules for Fire Safety

- Be sure matches and other fire risks are kept away from children.
- With patients who smoke, follow facility policy for smoking in the unit and supervise any patient not fully alert and mobile.
- Follow facility policy for posting "no smoking" signs and other preventive steps when oxygen is being used in the unit.
- Know the location of fire extinguishers and fire alarms and how to use them.
- Know what to do in your facility in case of fire; usually you should first remove any patients in immediate danger and then set off the alarm.
- Know the fire alarm code for your unit and others nearby.
- Never prop open fire doors.
- Close doors to patient rooms.
- Use extra care when working with flammable liquids such as some cleaning fluids.
- For children receiving oxygen, be sure there are no toys present that may cause sparks.

General Rules for Electrical Safety

- With children, use safety plugs in electrical outlets and keep cords and equipment out of reach.
- Before using electrical equipment, check carefully for a frayed cord or damaged outlet. If an electrical item is questionable, have it checked by the maintenance department.
- Avoid using a thin extension cord for equipment that has a heavier cord.

- Do not overload an outlet with more than two electrical appliances.
- Do not plug more than one piece of equipment into an extension cord.

General Rules for Using Restraints

- Physical patient restraints are used to prevent patients from falling out of bed or from a wheelchair, from interfering with equipment or dressings, or from harming themselves or others.
- Restrain a patient only when there is a clear doctor's order for the restraint--never just for convenience.
- Always apply restraints with great carefulness to prevent cutting off the patient's circulation or impairing breathing. Pad areas that may be injured.
- Provide frequent skin care to areas that are restrained.
- Check the restrained patient frequently, and reposition, offer a drink of water, offer a bedpan or urinal, and attend to all needs.
- Always explain to the patient and family members or visitors present that the restraint is being used for safety.
- Because the restrained patient may feel anger, humiliation, or confusion about the restraints, be especially sympathetic and supportive to the patient.
- A disoriented patient who is restrained may be slow to comprehend the restraints and need additional explanations and reassurance.

- Follow facility policy for reporting all information to the nurse and including information in the patient record.
- Always use the minimum amount of restraint that is effective for the individual patient; allow the patient some movement that will not allow removal of the restraints or any safety risks.
- Keep scissors nearby to cut a restraint free in an emergency.

PROCEDURE: APPLYING A SAFETY BELT

1. Ask another staff member for help if necessary.
2. Obtain a safety belt that will fit the patient.
3. Wash your hands.
4. Check the patient's identification bracelet and speak the patient's name.
5. Explain to the patient what you are doing..
6. Follow facility policy for asking visitors to leave the room.
7. Close the privacy curtain.
8. Locking arms with the patient, help the patient assume a sitting position.
9. Smooth the belt so that it is free of wrinkles.
10. Using one hand, position the belt on the patient's waist. With the other hand, pull the ties around to the patient's back.
11. Pull the ties through the slots.
12. Lock arms with the patient, and help the patient lie down in a comfortable position.
13. Tie the straps to the bed frame (never the side rails) using a square knot, or lock the straps if the belt locks. Be sure the knots or locks remain visible.

14. Make sure the patient can reach the signal light.
15. Open the privacy curtain.
16. Wash your hands.
17. Every 2 hours, remove the safety belt and provide skin care and motion exercises. Adjust the patient's position, and reapply the belt.
18. Report to the nurse that you have applied a safety belt to the patient.

PROCEDURE: APPLYING A JACKET RESTRAINT

1.   Ask another staff member for help if necessary.
2.   Obtain a jacket restraint that would fit the patient.
3.   Wash your hands.
4.   Check the patient's identification bracelet and speak the patient's name.
5.   Explain to the patient what you are doing.
6.   Follow facility policy for asking visitors to leave the room.
7.   Close the privacy curtain.
8.   Locking arms with the patient, help the patient assume a sitting position.
9.   With your free hand, place the patient's arms through the arm holes of the jacket. If the patient has an injured arm, place that arm through the arm hole first.
10. Smooth both the front and the back of the jacket, and cross the jacket panels in front.
11. Locking arms with the patient, help the patient lie down in a comfortable position.

12. Tie the straps to the bed frame using square knots, or lock the straps if the jacket locks. Be sure the knots or locks remain visible.
13. Make sure the patient can reach the signal light.
14. Open the privacy curtain.
15. Wash your hands.
16. Every 2 hours, remove the jacket and provide skin care and motion exercises. Adjust the patient's position, and reapply the jacket.
17. Report to the nurse that you have applied a safety jacket to the patient.

PROCEDURE: APPLYING MITT RESTRAINTS

1. Wash your hands.
2. Check the patient's identification bracelet and speak the patient's name.
3. Explain to the patient what you are doing.
4. Follow facility policy for asking visitors to leave the room.
5. Obtain 2 mitt restraints, 2 washcloths, a towel, and tape.
6. Close the privacy curtain.
7. Dry the patient's hands with the towel if they are moist.
8. To make a hand roll, fold a washcloth in half and roll it up. Use tape to keep the roll in place. Make a hand roll with each washcloth.
9. Place a hand roll in the patient's hand so that it rests naturally.
10. Put the mitt on the hand.
11. If the hand is to be immobilized, tie the straps to the bed frame using a square knot. Be sure the knot remains visible.

12. Restrain the other hand in the same way.
13. Make sure the patient can reach the signal light.
14. Open the privacy curtain.
15. Place the soiled towel in the laundry bag.
16. Wash your hands.
17. Every 2 hours, remove the mitts and provide skin care and motion exercises. Adjust the patient's position, and reapply the mitts.
18. Report to the nurse that you have applied mitt restraints to the patient's hands.

PROCEDURE: APPLYING ELBOW RESTRAINTS

Note: Elbow restraints are usually used with infants and young children to prevent scratching and touching of certain body areas.

1. Wash your hands.
2. Check the patient's identification bracelet and speak the patient's name.
3. Explain to the patient and parents, if present, what you are doing.
4. Follow facility policy for asking visitors to leave.
5. Obtain 2 elbow restraints, tongue depressors, and safety pins.
6. Close the privacy curtain.
7 To make the restraint rigid, insert the tongue depressors into the slots.
8. Wrap the restraint around the patient's elbow so that it is firm but comfortable.
9. Tie the strings around the patient's arm using square knots.

10. To prevent the restraint from sliding down the arm, pin the restraint to the patient's gown with the safety pins. Be sure the pins point down and away from the patient's body.
11. Restrain the other elbow in the same way.
12. Make sure the patient, or the patient's parents, can reach the signal light.
13. Open the privacy curtain.
14. Wash your hands.
15. Every 2 hours, remove the elbow restraints and provide skin care and motion exercises. Adjust the patient's position and reapply the elbow restraints.
16. Report to the nurse that you have restrained the patient's elbows.

PROCEDURE: APPLYING ANKLE AND WRIST RESTRAINTS

1. Wash your hands.
2. Check the patient's identification bracelet and speak the patient's name.
3. Explain to the patient what you are doing.
4. Follow facility policy for asking visitors to leave the room.
5. Obtain thick gauze dressings, roller bandage, and tape.
6. Close the privacy curtain.
7. Help the patient to assume a comfortable position.
8. Wrap the gauze dressing around the wrist or ankle, making sure it is secure but not tight. Tape the dressing in place.

9. To make a clove hitch, make a double loop with the roller bandage and pick up the loops together. Slip the patient's wrist or ankle through the two loops such that the loops are over the gauze dressing.
10. Tie the ends of the bandage to the bed frame using a square knot. Be sure the knot remains visible.
11. If so instructed, restrain the other wrists and ankles in the same way.
12. Make sure the patient can reach the signal light.
13. Open the privacy curtain.
14. Wash your hands.
15. Every 15 minutes, check the pulse, color, and temperature of any restrained wrist or ankle. Report to the nurse your observations.
16. Every 2 hours, remove the restraints and provide skin care and motion exercises. Adjust the patient's position, and reapply the restraints.
17. Report to the nurse that you have restrained the patient's wrists and ankles.

Chapter 3
Emergency Care

General Rules for Emergencies

- Always first call for help, following facility policy. Never assume the patient's condition will improve by itself or that you can give all the care needed by yourself.
- Stay calm; rushing in a panic disrupts the care process and frightens others present.

- If the patient is in a position of immediate danger, carefully move the patient only if you can without risk of danger to yourself.
- Do not start providing care until you have determined what is wrong.
- Look first for life-threatening problems: lack of breathing, blocked airway, lack of pulse, or severe bleeding. Care for these problems before doing anything else.
- Keep the patient warm and as comfortable as possible. Reassure the patient and explain everything you are doing.
- As trained, provide care for specific emergency problems (see following procedures).
- Prevent bystanders from crowding around the patient.
- Stay with the patient until medical help arrives.

PROCEDURE: PATIENT AFTER A FALL

1. Call for help.
2. Stay calm and do not try to do any procedure you have not been trained to do.
3. Do not move the patient.
4. Check for signs of injury: swelling, bruising, pain, bleeding, and unusual positioning of limbs.
5. Report signs of injury and all other facts to arriving help.
6. Stay with the patient until medical help arrives. Assist as directed in checking vital signs or moving the patient.

PROCEDURE: BLEEDING PATIENT

1. Call for help.
2. Stay calm and do not try to do any procedure you have not been trained to do.
3. Using disposable gloves and a clean cloth if available, put firm pressure on the wound with your hand.
4. If the bleeding is from an arm or leg, elevate the limb.
5. If the patient is standing, assist the patient to lie in bed or on the floor to prevent fainting.
6. Stay with the patient until medical help arrives.

PROCEDURE: PATIENT IN SHOCK

Note: The patient may be in shock if blood pressure is falling; the pulse is weak and rapid; the skin is cool, moist, and pale; breathing is rapid or shallow; and the patient is restless, anxious, or confused.

1. Call for help.
2. Stay calm and do not try to do any procedure you have not been trained to do.
3. Assist the patient to lie down, and raise the legs slightly if comfortable.
4. Keep the patient warm; cover with blanket if possible.
5. Check for and control any bleeding; do not move the patient if a bone may be broken.
6. Calm and reassure the patient.
7. Do not offer anything to drink.
8. Stay with the patient until medical help arrives.

PROCEDURE: PATIENT WITH STROKE

Note: The patient may have had a stroke if you observe unconsciousness or disorientation, difficult breathing, headache, paralysis of an arm or leg, difficulty in speaking or seeing, and/or convulsions.

1. Call for help.
2. Stay calm and do not try to do any procedure you have not been trained to do.
3. Be sure the patient's airway stays open.
4. Help the patient into a safe and comfortable position, being careful with paralyzed parts of the body.
5. Keep the patient warm.
6. Calm or reassure the patient.
7. Do not offer anything to drink.
8. Stay with the patient until medical help arrives.

PROCEDURE: PATIENT WITH HEART ATTACK

Note: The patient may have had a heart attack if you observe shortness of breath, difficult breathing, heavy sweating, cool, moist skin, nausea, pain in the chest and possibly in the left arm, neck, or jaw, and/or pale color.

1. Call for help.
2. Stay calm and do not try to do any procedure you have not been trained to do.
3. Help the patient into a comfortable position.
4. Loosen any tight clothing.
5. Calm or reassure the patient.
6. Carefully monitor breathing and pulse.
7. Do not offer anything to drink.

8. Stay with the patient until medical help arrives.

PROCEDURE: PATIENT WITH CARDIAC ARREST

Note: _The patient has cardiac arrest if the heart has stopped and there is no pulse. Other signs include unconsciousness, lack of breathing and bluish color of the lips and nailbeds._

1. Call for immediate and urgent help.
2. Stay calm and do not try to do any procedure you have not been trained to do.
3. Loosen any tight clothing.
4. ONLY if you have been trained in CPR, start CPR immediately. Otherwise, get help immediately.
5. Stay with the patient until medical help arrives.

PROCEDURE: PATIENT WITH SEIZURE

Note: _The patient may have had a seizure if you observe loss of consciousness followed by muscle contractions, clenched jaw, eyes rolled back, and jerking movements. The seizure will end by itself._

1. Call for help.
2. Stay calm and do not try to do any procedure you have not been trained to do.
3. Prevent the patient from becoming injured: lower the patient to the floor and put a pillow or other padding under the head.
4. Turn the patient's head to one side for saliva or vomit to drain from the mouth.
5. Loosen clothing.

6. Move any equipment the patient may bump
    into.
7. Do not try to restrain the patient's body
    movements.
8. Follow facility policy for inserting a padded
    tongue depressor between teeth ONLY if the
    teeth are not clenched.
9. Stay with the patient until medical help arrives.

PROCEDURE: PATIENT WHO FAINTED

1. Call for help.
2. Stay calm and do not try to do any procedure
    you have not been trained to do.
3. For a patient who feels about to faint, position
    the patient sitting with head bent forward
    between the knees or lying down with legs
    elevated.
4. Loosen any tight clothing.
5. Do not let the patient get up for several
    minutes after the symptoms are over.
6. Stay with the patient until medical help arrives.

PROCEDURE: BURNED PATIENT

1. Call for help.
2. Stay calm and do not try to do any procedure
    you have not been trained to do.
3. For a minor first degree burn (red skin only),
    put the burned part in cold water for several
    minutes and then cover with a clean dressing.
4. For a more serious burn, do not remove
    clothing stuck to the burned area but cover the
    area lightly with a clean damp cloth.
5. Stay with the patient until medical help arrives.

PROCEDURE: PATIENT AFTER POISONING

Note: _The patient may be experiencing poisoning if you observe an open container nearby, nausea and/or vomiting, irregular breathing, convulsions, unconsciousness or drowsiness, and/or burns around the mouth._

1. Call for help.
2. Stay calm and do not try to do any procedure you have not been trained to do.
3. Ask the patient about anything swallowed or inhaled, and look around the room for any signs of substances taken.
4. Away from the facility, call the poison control center (or 911) and follow their directions.
5. Monitor the patient's breathing, and if trained, give CPR if the patient stops breathing.
6. Keep the patient warm and comfortable.
7. Stay with the patient until medical help arrives.

PROCEDURE: OPENING THE AIRWAY– CONSCIOUS ADULT OR CHILD

1. Call for help.
2. Stay calm and do not try to do any procedure you have not been trained to do.
3. Confirm the patient is choking by asking the patient, "Can you speak?"
4. Perform abdominal thrusts (Heimlich maneuver) to clear the airway:
    a. Stand behind the patient.
    b. Put your arms around the victim's waist.

    c. Make a fist of one hand and put the thumb side against the abdomen below the breastbone.

    d. Grasp your fist with the other hand and give a quick upward thrust into the patient's abdomen.

    e. Give separate thrusts, one after another, until the airway clears or the patient becomes unconscious (see next procedure).

5. Stay with the patient until medical help arrives.

PROCEDURE: OPENING THE AIRWAY-- UNCONSCIOUS ADULT OR CHILD

1. Call for help.
2. Stay calm and do not try to do any procedure you have not been trained to do.
3. Position the patient lying on the back.
4. Check to see if the patient is breathing.
5. Open the airway by tilting the head back and lifting the chin. If there is any danger of a neck injury, do not tilt the head back.
6. If you have been trained in rescue breathing, pinch the patient's nose shut and give two full breaths. If the breaths cannot go into the patient, perform abdominal thrusts to open the airway.
7. To perform abdominal thrusts:
    a. Turn the patient's head to one side.
    b. Kneel next to or straddle the patient's thighs.
    c. Put the heel of one hand on the patient's abdomen below the bottom of the

  breastbone. Put your other hand on top of
  the first.
  d. Give a thrust by pressing inward and
   upward. Repeat up to 10 times.
8. Sweep the patient's mouth with your finger to
  remove any dislodged object.
  a. With one hand put your thumb into the
   mouth and grasp and lift both the lower jaw
   and tongue to open mouth fully.
  b. Use index finger of other hand along inside
   of cheek and deep to base of tongue to
   hook out any object. Be careful not to
   push an object deeper into the mouth or
   throat.
  c. Remove the object.
9. If patient is still not breathing, give two full
  breaths. If airway is still blocked, repeat
  abdominal thrusts (step 7) and finger sweep
  (step 8) continually until the airway clears or
  help arrives.
10. Stay with the patient until medical help arrives.

PROCEDURE: OPENING THE AIRWAY-- CONSCIOUS INFANT

1. Call for help.
2. Stay calm and do not try to do any procedure
  you have not been trained to do.
3. Confirm that the infant's airway is blocked.
4. Perform back blows:
  a. With one hand supporting the infant's neck
   and chest, hold infant face down over your
   thigh, with head below body level.

    b. With the heel of the other hand, give 4 blows to the infant's back between the shoulder blades.

5.   If the airway does not clear, perform chest thrusts:

    a. Turn the infant face up on your thigh, with head lower than trunk.

    b. Position hand on infant's chest in same place as for CPR (see following procedure).

    c. Give 4 chest thrusts 4 seconds apart.

6.   If the object has not dislodged, repeat alternating back blows and chest thrusts until the airway clears or the infant loses consciousness.

7.   Stay with the patient until medical help arrives.

PROCEDURE: OPENING THE AIRWAY--UNCONSCIOUS INFANT

1.   Call for help.

2.   Stay calm and do not try to do any procedure you have not been trained to do.

3.   Confirm that the infant is not breathing and unconscious.

4.   Position the infant face up on a hard flat surface.

5.   Tilt the infant's head back and lift its chin, being careful not to hyperextend the neck.

6.   If not breathing, give one rescue breath. If the breath will not go in, reposition the infant and try with another breath.

7. Perform back blows:
    a. With one hand supporting the infant's neck
       and chest, hold infant face down over your
       thigh, with head below body level.
    b. With the heel of the other hand, give 4
       blows to the infant's back between the
       shoulder blades.
8. If the airway does not clear, perform chest
    thrusts:
    a. Turn the infant face up on your thigh, with
       head lower than trunk.
    b. Position hand on infant's chest in same
       place as for CPR (see following procedure).
    c. Give 4 chest thrusts 4 seconds apart.
9. Check the infant's mouth to remove any
    dislodged object.
    a. With one hand put your thumb into the
       mouth and grasp and lift both the lower jaw
       and tongue to open mouth fully.
    b. Only if you see a foreign object use index
       finger of other hand to hook it out. Be
       careful not to push an object deeper into
       the mouth or throat.
10. Open the airway by tilting the head back and
    lifting the chin. Check for breathing. Try to
    give one breath to the infant.
11. If the airway is still blocked, continue the steps
    for back blows, chest thrusts, and mouth
    check until the airway clears or help arrives.
12. Stay with the patient until medical help arrives.

PROCEDURE: CPR FOR ADULT

Note: *CPR (cardiopulmonary resuscitation) is used for patients whose heart and breathing both have stopped, such as may happen after a severe heart attack or with many other conditions.*

1. Call for immediate and urgent help.
2. Stay calm and do not try to do any procedure you have not been trained to do. NEVER ATTEMPT TO PERFORM CPR UNLESS YOU HAVE PASSED A CPR COURSE.
3. Confirm the patient is unconscious.
4. Position the patient on the back on a hard flat surface.
5. Open the airway by tilting the head back and lifting the chin.
6. Check to see if the patient is breathing. If not breathing, pinch nose closed and give two full breaths to the patient, pausing in between.
7. Confirm that the patient's chest rises and falls with the breaths. If not, reposition to open the airway and if needed clear an obstruction with abdominal thrusts (see earlier procedure).
8. Confirm that there is no pulse. Feel for the carotid pulse for 5-10 seconds.
9. Position hands to give chest compressions:
   a. Locate lower edge of ribs using your hand closest to the patient's legs.
   b. Slide your fingers up the edge of the rib cage to the notch at the lower end of the breastbone.
   c. Put your middle finger in the notch and the index finger beside it just above the end of the breastbone.

    d. Place the heel of your other hand on the breastbone next to the positioned index finger.

    e. Place the heel of the first hand on top of the positioned hand on the breastbone. Keep fingers off the chest.

10. Position yourself so that your shoulders are over your hands, with your arms straight and elbows locked.

11. Give 15 chest compressions:

    a. With each, compress the breastbone 1.5 to 2 inches.

    b. Compress at a rate of 80 to 100 compressions per minute.

    c. Compress smoothly up and down with hands always in contact with chest.

12. After 15 compressions open the airway and give 2 full breaths.

13. Complete a total of 4 cycles of 2 breaths and 15 compressions.

14. Feel for a carotid pulse for 5 seconds.

15. If no pulse, continue the cycle of giving 2 breaths and 15 compressions. Every few minutes check for a pulse.

16. If the patient's pulse starts, check for breathing. Continue rescue breathing if needed.

17. If the pulse does not start, continue CPR until help arrives.

18. Stay with the patient until medical help arrives.

PROCEDURE: CPR FOR INFANT OR CHILD

1. Call for immediate and urgent help.
2. Stay calm and do not try to do any procedure you have not been trained to do. NEVER ATTEMPT TO PERFORM CPR UNLESS YOU HAVE PASSED A CPR COURSE.
3. Confirm the patient is unconscious.
4. Position the patient on the back on a hard flat surface. Support the head and neck while turning.
5. Open the airway by tilting the head back and lifting the chin. With an infant be careful not to hyperextend the neck.
6. Check to see if the patient is breathing. If not breathing, give two full slow breaths to the patient, pausing in between. With an infant, cover the nose and mouth with your mouth; with a child, pinch the nose closed and breathe in through the mouth.
7. Confirm that the patient's chest rises and falls with the breaths. If not, reposition to open the airway and if needed clear an obstruction (see earlier procedure).
8. Confirm that there is no pulse. Feel for 5-10 seconds. Use the carotid pulse for children and the brachial pulse for infants.
9. Give chest compressions:
   For child:
   a. Locate lower edge of ribs using your hand closest to the patient's legs.
   b. Slide your fingers up the edge of the rib cage to the notch at the lower end of the breastbone.

c. Put your middle finger in the notch and the index finger beside it just above the end of the breastbone.
d. Place the heel of your other hand on the breastbone next to the positioned index finger.
e. Place the heel of the first hand on top of the positioned hand on the breastbone. Keep fingers off the chest.
f. Position yourself so that your shoulders are over your hands, with your arms straight and elbows locked.
g. For each compression, compress the breastbone 1.5 to 2 inches.
h. Compress at a rate of 80 to 100 compressions per minute.
i. Compress smoothly up and down with hands always in contact with chest.

For infant:
a. Imagine a line drawn between the infant's nipples.
b. Using the hand farther from the infant's head, put your index finger in the middle of the chest just below this line.
c. Position your middle and ring fingers beside the index finger. The compression area is beneath these two fingers.
d. For each compression, compress the breastbone 0.5 to 1 inch.
e. Compress at a rate of 100 compressions per minute.
f. Compress smoothly, releasing pressure after each but not removing hand from the chest.

10. After 5 compressions open the airway and give 1 full breath.
11. Complete a total of 10 cycles of 5 compressions and 1 breath.
14. Feel for a pulse for 5 seconds.
15. If no pulse, continue the cycle of giving 1 breath and 5 compressions. Every few minutes check for a pulse.
16. If the patient's pulse starts, check for breathing. Continue rescue breathing if needed.
17. If the pulse does not start, continue CPR until help arrives.
18. Stay with the patient until medical help arrives.

Chapter 4
The Patient in the Unit

This chapter includes information on the following:

Principles for the Unit

► Make sure the unit is always safe and clean.
► Make sure the patient can always reach the signal light, the overbed table and personal possessions, water glass and pitcher (if not NPO), the telephone, and television and other controls.
► Be sure the patient has sufficient tissues, toilet paper, and personal toiletries.
► Make sure the unit's temperature and lighting are comfortable for the patient.
► Explain any equipment in the room to the patient.
► Help control odors and noise in the room; explain any unusual factors to the patient.
► Frequently empty the wastepaper basket.
► Adjust the privacy curtain to the patient's preference; always use the privacy curtain when giving care.
► Always be courteous and friendly to the patient, family, and visitors.

Principles for Furniture and Equipment

- ▸ Use the lowest horizontal bed position when the patient is getting in or out of bed, and a raised position to provide patient care with good body mechanics.
- ▸ With electric beds, teach patients how to use controls and which positions to use.
- ▸ Be sure bed wheels are locked in place when the patient gets in or out of bed and when giving care.
- ▸ Always use special bed equipment such as a bed board or bed cradle exactly as ordered.
- ▸ Adjust the height of the overbed table for the patient's comfort when eating, writing, and so on.
- ▸ When using the overbed table as a working area, put only clean equipment and supplies on the table surface; wash the surface after using it.
- ▸ Unit chairs can be used temporarily to hold supplies such as clean bed linens but not dirty equipment or supplies.
- ▸ Be sure the bathroom is kept clean and is always stocked with appropriate supplies.
- ▸ Always follow facility policy for use of special equipment in the unit, giving attention to safety factors.
- ▸ Follow facility policy for the use of disposable equipment and supplies, some of which are used only once but others are used repeatedly but only for the same patient.

General Rules for Admitting Patients

- During admission the admission record is completed with all patient data, the identification bracelet is put on the patient's wrist, and the patient signs a consent form for treatment.
- Because the patient and family are often fearful or worried, all nursing staff should be friendly and courteous.
- Always greet the patient by name, and introduce yourself as well to family members and friends.
- Use the facility's admission checklist completely and carefully.

PROCEDURE: PREPARING THE ROOM FOR THE PATIENT

1. Confirm the room and bed to be prepared.
2. Wash your hands.
3. Be sure the patient admission pack is present with personal care items.
4. Check that all unit equipment such as the bedpan is present and in place.
5. Place the overbed table on the right side for a right-handed patient or on the left for a left-handed patient.
6. Place the signal cord on the right side for a right-handed patient or on the left for a left-handed patient.
7. If appropriate, close privacy curtains or screen.
8. Open the bed.
9. Wash your hands.

PROCEDURE: ADMITTING THE PATIENT

1. Wash your hands.
2. Confirm the room is prepared and all appropriate equipment present.
3. Introduce yourself to the patient in a friendly way. Ask for the name the patient prefers to use. Explain your title and role in providing care.
4. If a roommate or other staff are present, introduce the patient.
5. Care for the patient's valuables following facility policy. Arrange personal items on the bedside table.
6. Ask family members and visitors to leave, if that is policy, while you finish admission.
7. Provide privacy by closing the room door and/or privacy curtains.
8. Ask the patient to change into a gown or pajamas. Help the patient if necessary (see Chapter 7). Hang clothes in the closet.
9. Measure the patient's height and weight (see following procedure).
10. Position the patient comfortably in the bed or bedside chair, as the nurse orders. Arrange the bed linens to the patient's comfort.
11. Raise the bed side rails if appropriate.
12. Complete your facility's admission checklist fully and accurately. Take vital signs if appropriate.
13. If the patient is allowed to have drinking water, fill the pitcher and position it within reach.
14. If the facility's policy is to obtain a urine specimen, explain this to the patient and assist the patient if needed (see Chapter 11).

15. Show the patient how to work the call signal and position the cord within easy reach.
16. Show the patient how to work the TV remote control, if present.
17. Explain how to use the telephone for outside calls. Position the telephone within easy reach.
18. Explain facility policies regarding visiting hours, meals, mail, and so on.
19. Explain what services are available to the patient, such as activities, programs, religious services, and so on.
20. Lower the bed. If allowed for the patient, elevate the head of the bed for the patient's comfort. If the patient can adjust the bed, show how to use the controls.
21. Unless the patient requests privacy, draw back the curtains.
22. Raise bed side rails if ordered or necessary for safety.
23. Double-check the call light is within easy reach.
24. Ask if the patient needs anything else.
25. Wash your hands.
26. Report to the nurse that you have completed the admission and any observations about the patient.

PROCEDURE: MEASURING HEIGHT AND WEIGHT

1. Wash your hands.
2. Check the patient's identification bracelet and speak the patient's name.

3. Explain to the patient what you are going to do.
4. Follow facility policy for asking visitors to leave the room.
5. Collect the following equipment: portable balance scale, paper and pen, paper towels. Balance the scale before beginning.
6. Close the privacy curtain.
7. Cover the scale platform with paper towels.
8. Ask the patient to remove robe, slippers, and any other clothing except gown or pajamas.
9. Help the patient to stand with both feet on the scale platform, with arms at the sides.
10. Slide the scale weights until the balance pointer is in the middle.
11. Write down the patient's name and weight.
12. Raise the height measuring rod over the patient's head.
13. Make sure the patient is standing straight, and lower the measurement rod until it rests on the patient's head.
14. Write down the patient's height.
15. Raise the measuring rod and help the patient off the scale.
16. Assist the patient to dress again or return to bed.
17. Make sure the patient can reach the signal light.
18. Discard used paper towels and return the scale.
19. Open the privacy curtain.
20. Wash your hands.
21. Report to the nurse that you have weighed and measured the patient and any unusual observations.

22. Record the measurements in the appropriate place.

PROCEDURE: TRANSFERRING THE PATIENT TO ANOTHER UNIT

1. Confirm where the patient is going and that the new unit is ready.
2. Check what method of transfer will be used to move the patient.
3. Obtain a wheelchair or stretcher and cart.
4. Wash your hands.
5. Check the patient's identification bracelet and speak the patient's name.
6. Explain to the patient what you are going to do.
7. Put on the cart the patient's personal belongings and equipment that are to be transferred.
8. Help the patient onto the stretcher or into the wheelchair (see Chapter 6).
9. Transport the patient to the new unit, following facility safety policies.
10. If present, introduce the patient to a roommate or receiving staff.
11. Help the receiving staff to position the patient.
12. Bring the patient's belongings to the new unit on the cart and arrange or put them away.
13. Make sure the patient is settled in the new unit, with bed properly adjusted, privacy curtain open, and signal light within the patient's reach.
14. Return the wheelchair or stretcher and cart to their storage places.
15. Wash your hands.

16. Report to the nurse the transfer and any unusual observations.
17. According to your responsibilities, return to the original unit and strip the bed and clean the unit.

PROCEDURE: DISCHARGING THE PATIENT

1. Confirm that the patient is to be discharged and that transportation has been arranged.
2. Wash your hands.
3. Check the patient's identification bracelet and speak the patient's name.
4. Explain to the patient what you are going to do.
5. Collect a wheelchair, a cart if needed for the patient's possessions, and the discharge slip.
6. Help the patient gather and pack all personal belongings. Check drawers and closets.
7. Follow facility policy for confirming the patient has all clothing and personal possessions.
8. If needed, help the patient dress (see Chapter 7).
9. Be sure the patient has written discharge instructions including any prescriptions, doctor's orders, and future appointments.
10. Move the wheelchair to the bedside and lock the wheels. Help the patient into the wheelchair. Unlock the wheels.
11. Follow facility policy to wheel the patient to a discharge desk, business office, or exit area. Complete the discharge slip or release form.
12. In the exit area lock the wheels and help the patient out of the wheelchair and into the car. Assist with belongings.

13. Return the wheelchair and cart to the storage area.
14. Wash your hands.
15. Report to the nurse the time of discharge, the transportation method, who accompanied the patient, and any observations.
16. If included in your responsibilities, return to the unit and strip the bed and clean the unit.

Chapter 5
Bedmaking

This chapter includes information on the following:
General rules for making beds
Procedure: Making a closed bed
Procedure: Making an occupied bed
Procedure: Making an open or empty bed
Procedure: Making a surgical bed

General Rules for Making Beds

- Wash your hands after handling soiled bed linens and before touching clean linens.
- Never shake bed linen, which may spread germs.
- Unused linen brought into a patient's room is considered contaminated and cannot be used somewhere else.
- Do not let either dirty or clean linen touch your uniform.
- Put dirty linen in the laundry bag, never on the floor even temporarily.
- Be sure the bottom sheet is free of wrinkles, which can cause discomfort and bed sores.
- If a plastic drawsheet is used, be sure it is covered with a cotton drawsheet to prevent the patient from touching the plastic.
- To save time and your energy, make as much of the bed as you can on one side before going to the other side.
- Always follow the policies of your institution for handling clean and dirty linen.

PROCEDURE: MAKING A CLOSED BED

1. Wash your hands.
2. Collect clean linen: mattress pad, bottom sheet, cotton and plastic drawsheets, top sheet, blanket, bedspread, pillowcase, and pillow.
3. Place the linen on a chair next to the bed, preferably on the side near the door.
4. Raise the bed to a high level to ease your body movements, and lock the bed wheels in place.
5. Pull the mattress to the head of the bed.
6. Place the mattress pad on the mattress, making sure that the pad touches the head of the mattress.
7. Fold the bottom sheet lengthwise and place the center crease in the middle of the mattress. Make sure the hem stitching faces the mattress. Position the sheet's short hem to hang over the bottom edge of the mattress and the longer hem to hang the same amount over the mattress's top edge.
8. Open the sheet and let the long edges hang the same distance over each side.
9. Tuck the top of the sheet smoothly and tightly under the mattress head.
10. Make a hospital (mitered) corner on one side. Pick up the side edge of the sheet 12 inches from the head of the bed. Raise the sheet onto the mattress. Tuck the remaining portion of the sheet under the mattress. Holding the fold at the edge of the mattress, lower the raised portion of the sheet. Tightly tuck the entire side of the sheet under the mattress.

11. Standing on the same side, fold the plastic drawsheet lengthwise and place it about 14 inches from the head of the bed.
12. Open the plastic sheet and tuck it in tightly.
13. Open the cotton drawsheet and cover the plastic sheet entirely with it. Tightly tuck the cotton drawsheet under the mattress.
14. Moving to the other side of the bed, make a hospital corner at the head of the bottom sheet.
15. Pulling to prevent wrinkles, tuck the bottom sheet under the mattress.
16. Pulling to prevent wrinkles, tuck both the plastic and cotton drawsheets under the mattress.
17. Returning to the other side of the bed, fold the top sheet lengthwise and place the center crease in the middle of the bed.
18. Place the large hem even with the top edge of the mattress and with the hem stitching facing out.
19. Open the sheet and let the long edges hang the same distance over each side. Do not tuck it in yet.
20. Fold the blanket lengthwise and place the center crease on the middle of the bed, leaving 6 inches from the top of the mattress. Open the blanket and let the long edges hang the same distance over each side. Do not tuck it in yet.
21. Fold the bedspread lengthwise and place the center crease on the middle of the bed, placing the upper hem even with the top of the mattress. Open the bedspread and let the

long edges hang the same distance over each
side.

22. Pulling the linens smooth and tight, tuck in the
top sheet, blanket, and bedspread at the foot
of the bed. Make a hospital corner on each
side of the bed.

23. Move to the head of the bed, and fold the top
hem of the bedspread under the top hem of
the blanket. Fold the top hem of the top sheet
back over the edge of the bedspread and
blanket to form a cuff. Smooth the top sheet
down over the bedspread.

24. Place the pillowcase flat on the bed.

25. Pick up the pillow, holding the two corners at
the tag end with one hand. Open the
pillowcase with your other hand. Insert the
pillow into the pillowcase until the end is
reached. Release the pillow corners, letting
them fall into corners of the case. Fold extra
pillowcase material under the pillow at the
seam end of the case.

26. Place the pillow on the bed with the pillowcase
seam facing the head of the bed and with the
pillow's open end facing away from the door.

27. Lower the bed to its lowest horizontal position,
and lock the bed wheels in place.

28. Wash your hands.

PROCEDURE: MAKING AN OCCUPIED BED

1. Wash your hands.
2. Check the patient's identification bracelet and
speak the patient's name.
3. Follow facility policy for asking visitors to leave
the room.

4. Explain to the patient that you are going to make the bed and how to help.
5. Close the privacy curtain.
6. Collect clean linen: bath blanket, mattress pad, bottom sheet, plastic and cotton drawsheets, top sheet, blanket, pillowcase, pillow, laundry bag.
7. Place the linen on a chair next to the bed.
8. Remove the call signal from the bed.
9. Raise the bed to a high level to ease your body movements.
10. Lower the backrest and kneerest to the flattest level that is comfortable for the patient, and lock the bed wheels in place.
11. Lower the side rail on the side you will work on. Raise the other side rail.
12. Loosen the top linens around the entire bed.
13. Remove the bedspread and blanket separately. Put them in the laundry bag if they are to be replaced, or fold them and place them on the chair if they are to be reused.
14. Cover the patient by placing the bath blanket over the top sheet. Ask the patient to hold the bath blanket. If the patient cannot do so, tuck the top edges of the bath blanket under the shoulders. Reaching under the bath blanket, grasp the top edge of the top sheet. Pull the top sheet down to the foot of the bed, and remove it. Put it in the linen bag.
15. Move the mattress to the head of the bed.
16. Ask the patient to turn on the side toward the far side of the bed, helping as necessary. Adjust the pillow on the far side of the bed. If the patient cannot sit up, lock arms at the

shoulder to raise the head and shoulders. Slide the pillow out and adjust it under the patient's head.

17. Fold the bottom linens separately toward the patient and tuck them against the back. Start with the cotton drawsheet, and then fold the plastic drawsheet and bottom sheet.

18. If the mattress pad is to be replaced, fold a clean mattress pad lengthwise and place the crease in the center of the bed. Fold the top part toward the patient. If the existing mattress pad is clean and can be reused, smooth out any wrinkles.

19. Fold the clean bottom sheet lengthwise and place the crease in the middle of the bed. The hem stitching should face the mattress, and the smaller hem should be even with the foot of the mattress. Fold the top half toward the patient's back.

20. Make a hospital (mitered) corner at the head of the bed. Tuck in the clean bottom sheet along the length of the bed.

21. If the plastic drawsheet is to be replaced, fold a clean plastic drawsheet lengthwise and place the crease in the center of the bed. Fold the top part toward the patient, and tuck in the hanging edges along the length of the bed. If the existing plastic drawsheet can be reused, pull it over the clean bottom sheet and tuck it in.

22. Fold the clean cotton drawsheet in half lengthwise, and cover the plastic drawsheet with it. Fold the top part toward the patient, and tuck in the hanging edges along the length of the bed.

23. Raise the bed rail on your side of the bed and lock it in place.
24. Move to the other side of the bed and lower the bed rail.
25. Ask the patient to roll over the linens in the center of the bed, helping if necessary. Move the pillow under the head.
26. Remove separately the soiled bottom sheet and cotton drawsheet and, if necessary, the soiled mattress pad and plastic drawsheet. Put all soiled linens in the laundry bag.
27. Smooth the mattress pad.
28. Pull the clean bottom sheet toward the edge of the bed. Make a hospital corner at the head of the bed, and tuck in the bottom sheet along the length of the bed. Pull tightly to remove wrinkles.
29. Pull the plastic and cotton drawsheets toward you tightly. Tuck each drawsheet under the mattress separately, smoothing out any wrinkles.
30. Ask the patient to turn on the back, helping if necessary. Adjust the pillow under the patient's head.
31. Spread the clean top sheet over the bath blanket, positioning the center crease in the middle of the bed. The wide hem should be at the head of the bed, and the hem stitching should face away from the patient.
32. Ask the patient to hold the top sheet. If the patient cannot do so, tuck the top edges under the shoulders. Reach under the top sheet and grasp the top edge of the bath blanket. Pull the bath blanket down toward the foot of the

bed. Remove it and discard in the laundry bag.

33. Spread the clean blanket over the top sheet, positioning the center crease in the middle of the bed. The top edge should be 6 inches from the top of the bed, or high enough to cover the patient's shoulders.

34. Spread the clean bed spread over the blanket, positioning the center crease in the middle of the bed. The top hem should be even with the edge of the mattress.

35. Move to the head of the bed, and fold the top hem of the bedspread over the top hem of the blanket. Fold the top hem of the top sheet back over the edges of the bedspread and blanket to form a cuff. Make sure the stitched hem of the top sheet faces away from the patient.

36. Move to the foot of the bed. Raising the mattress corner with one arm, tuck the top sheet, blanket, and bedspread under the mattress. Make sure the patient has enough room to move the feet comfortably. Make a hospital corner on each side.

37. Raise the side rail. Smooth the top linens.

38. Remove the pillow from beneath the patient's head. If necessary, lock arms at the shoulder to raise the head and shoulders, then slide the pillow out. Remove the soiled pillowcase and put it in the laundry bag. Put a clean pillowcase on the pillow, and place the pillow under the patient's head.

39. Attach the signal light so that the patient can reach it.

40. Lower the bed to its lowest horizontal position.

41. Raise the backrest and kneerest to safe and comfortable levels.
42. Open the privacy curtain.
43. Move the overbed table into a position within easy reach of the patient.
44. Make sure all soiled linen is in the linen bag, and place the bag in the dirty utility room or in the laundry chute.
45. Wash your hands.

PROCEDURE: MAKING AN OPEN BED

1. Wash your hands.
2. Stand on one side of your equipment, a closed bed.
3. Grasp the cuff of the top linens in both hands, and fold the linens to the foot of the bed.
4. So a patient can more easily grasp the bedding, fold the top linens back toward the head of the bed. The edge of the cuff should meet the fold.
5. Smooth the top and hanging sides of the linens.
6. Attach the signal light within a patient's reach.
7. Lower the bed to its lowest horizontal position.
8. Wash your hands.

PROCEDURE: MAKING A SURGICAL BED

1. Wash your hands.
2. Collect clean equipment: mattress pad, bottom sheet, plastic and cotton drawsheets, top sheet, blanket, pillowcase, pillow, bedspread, laundry bag, tissue box, emesis basin, IV pole.

3. Place the linen on a chair next to the bed.
4. Raise the bed to a high level to ease your body movements, and lock the bed wheels in place.
5. Remove the call signal from the bed.
6. Strip the bed of all used linen, placing it in the laundry bag.
7. Following the instructions for making a closed bed, make the bottom part of the bed.
8. Following the instructions for making a closed bed, make the top part of the bed. Do not tuck in the top linens.
9. Fold all the linens at the foot of the bed back onto the bed. The folded edge should be even with the edge of the mattress.
10. Fold the top linens back so that the patient can easily be transferred to the bed. Either fold the top linens lengthwise toward the side away from the door, or fold the top linens down from the head of the bed to the foot.
11. Put a clean pillowcase on the pillow.
12. Position the pillow against the headboard to protect the patient's head.
13. Adjust the bed to its highest horizontal position, and lower both side rails.
14. Move all furniture away from the bed to make room for the stretcher.
15. Place the tissue box and emesis basin on the bedside table, and clear away any other objects.
16. Place an IV pole near the head of the bed.
17. Make sure all soiled linen is in the linen bag, and place the bag in the dirty utility room or in the laundry chute.
18. Wash your hands.

Chapter 6
Lifting and Moving Patients

This chapter includes information on the following:

*Procedure: Moving the patient from stretcher to
    bed*
Procedure: Using a mechanical lift

Principles of Body Mechanics

- Keep your body aligned while performing all
  procedures: back straight, feet apart, knees
  slightly bent.
- When lifting or carrying objects, keep them
  close to your body.
- If possible, push or slide a heavy object rather
  than lifting it.
- To lift an object, never bend over but squat to
  grasp it and use the leg muscles rather than
  back muscles to raise yourself.
- Distribute weight and effort among your
  muscles; use both hands instead of one for
  heavy objects.
- Always position your body facing the task being
  performed; avoid twisting your body.
- Ask a coworker for help when moving heavy
  objects or patients; count one, two, three with
  the coworker to coordinate your movements.

General Rules for Moving the Patient

- Always make sure first that the patient has no
  restrictions on movements or positions.
- Always first explain to the patient what you are
  about to do and how the patient can help.
- Always consider first whether you need help
  from coworkers before you start to move the
  patient.
- Be careful to prevent the patient from becoming
  uncovered or exposed during movement.

- Maintain good body alignment at all times and follow the principles of body mechanics (see above).
- When holding the patient during movement, keep the patient's body close to yours.
- Before starting to move a patient, watch for and protect any tubing, drainage containers, ostomy appliances, and other equipment attached to the patient.

PROCEDURE: LOCKING ARMS WITH THE PATIENT

1. Wash your hands.
2. Check the patient's identification bracelet and speak the patient's name.
3. Explain that you are going to raise the patient by locking arms.
4. Follow facility policy for asking visitors to leave the room.
5. Close the privacy curtain.
6. Lock the bed wheels, and raise the bed to a high level to ease your body movements.
7. Lower only the near side rail.
8. Face the head of the bed, and ask the patient to put the arm nearest you under your near arm. The patient's hand should reach up your back and rest on your shoulder. (Depending on which side you are standing, the patient's right hand will be on your right shoulder, or the left hand will be on your left shoulder.)
9. To lock arms, put your near arm under the patient's near arm, and put your hand on the patient's shoulder.

10. Use your free hand to support the patient's neck and shoulders from behind.
11. On your count of three, help the patient assume a sitting position.
12. Use your free hand to adjust linens, gown, or pillow.
13. Help the patient lie down by supporting the body with your locked arm and by supporting the neck and shoulders with your free arm.
14. Lower the bed to a comfortable and safe position.
15. Raise the side rail.
16. Make sure the patient can reach the signal light.
17. Open the privacy curtain.
18. Wash your hands.

PROCEDURE: MOVING THE PATIENT UP IN BED WITH PATIENT'S HELP

1. Wash your hands.
2. Check the patient's identification bracelet and speak the patient's name.
3. Explain that you are going to move the patient up in bed and how he can help.
4. Follow facility policy for asking visitors to leave the room.
5. Close the privacy curtain.
6. Lock the bed wheels, and raise the bed to a high level to ease your body movements.
7. Lower the headrest to the lowest horizontal position that is safe for the patient.
8. To prevent head injury, place the pillow against the headboard.
9. Lower only the near side rail.

10. Facing the head of the bed, stand with your feet about 12 inches apart. Point the foot closest to the head of the bed in that direction.
11. Keeping your back straight, bend your knees.
12. Ask the patient to bend the knees, reach backward, and grasp the head of the bed.
13. Position one arm under the patient's thighs and the other under the shoulders.
14. On your count of three, have the patient pull with the hands toward the head of the bed and push with the feet against the mattress. At the same time, slide the patient's body with your hands and arms to the desired place.
15. Lock arms with the patient, and slip the pillow under the head and shoulders. Smooth the bed linens.
16. Raise the headrest to a safe and comfortable position.
17. Lower the bed to its lowest horizontal position.
18. Raise the side rail.
19. Make sure the patient can reach the signal light.
20. Open the privacy curtain.
21. Wash your hands.

PROCEDURE: MOVING THE PATIENT UP IN BED WITH ASSISTANT

1. Ask a nursing assistant to help you.
2. Wash your hands.
3. Check the patient's identification bracelet and speak the patient's name.
4. Explain that you and the other assistant are going to help the patient move up in bed.

5. Follow facility policy for asking visitors to leave the room.
6. Close the privacy curtain.
7. Lock the bed wheels, and raise the bed to a high level to ease your body movements.
8. Lower the headrest to the lowest horizontal position that is safe for the patient.
9. To prevent head injury, place the pillow against the headboard.
10. Stand on one side of the bed and ask your partner to stand on the other side. Lower the side rails.
11. Facing the head of the bed, you and your partner should stand broadly with your feet about 12 inches apart. Point the foot closest to the head of the bed in that direction.
12. Keeping your back straight, bend your knees.
13. Position one arm under the patient's buttocks and the other under the shoulders. Your partner should do the same. Join forearms with your partner.
14. Ask the patient to bend both knees. Ask the patient if possible to help by pushing the feet against the bed on your count of three.
15. On your count of three, slide the patient's body with your hands and arms to the desired place. You and your partner should move together.
16. Lock arms with the patient, and slip the pillow under the patient's head and shoulders. Smooth the bed linens.
17. Raise the headrest to a safe and comfortable position.
18. Lower the bed to its lowest horizontal position.
19. Raise the side rails.

20. Make sure the patient can reach the signal light.
21. Open the privacy curtain.
22. Wash your hands.

PROCEDURE: MOVING THE PATIENT TO SIDE OF BED

1. Wash your hands.
2. Check the patient's identification bracelet and speak the patient's name.
3. Explain that you are going to move the patient to the side of the bed and how he can help.
4. Follow facility policy for asking visitors to leave the room.
5. Close the privacy curtain.
6. Lock the bed wheels, and raise the bed to a high level to ease your body movements.
7. Lower the headrest to the lowest horizontal level that is safe for the patient.
8. Stand on the side of the bed to which the patient will be moved.
9. Lower the near side rail, and make sure the far side rail is raised.
10. Loosen the top sheets.
11. Cross the patient's arms over the chest.
12. Stand broadly with your feet about 12 inches apart. Keeping your back straight, bend your knees.
13. Slide one arm under the patient's shoulders and hold the far shoulder. Slide the other arm under the middle of the back.
14. Rocking back onto your rear foot, move the patient's upper body toward you.

15. Slide one arm under the patient's waist and the other arm under the thighs.
16. Rocking back onto your rear foot, move the patient's body toward you.
17. Slide one arm under the patient's thighs and the other arm under the feet.
18. Rocking back onto your rear foot, move the patient's legs and feet toward you.
19. Lock arms with the patient, and slip the pillow under the patient's head and shoulders. Smooth the bed linens.
20. Raise the headrest to a safe and comfortable position.
21. Lower the bed to its lowest horizontal position.
22. Raise the side rail.
23. Make sure the patient can reach the signal light.
24. Open the privacy curtain.
25. Wash your hands.

PROCEDURE: HELPING THE PATIENT SIT ON THE SIDE OF BED

1. Wash your hands.
2. Check the patient's identification bracelet and speak the patient's name.
3. Explain that you are going to help the patient sit on the side of the bed.
4. Follow facility policy for asking visitors to leave the room.
5. Obtain the patient's robe and slippers, a sheet, and a footstool if the patient is short.
6. Close the privacy curtain.
7. If necessary, move furniture so that you and the patient can move easily.

8. Lock the bed wheels, and raise the bed to a high level to ease your body movements.
9. Lower the headrest to the lowest level that is safe for the patient.
10. Help the patient move up in bed.
11. Fold the top linens down to the foot of the bed. Place the sheet under the patient's feet, and put the slippers on the patient.
12. Help the patient move to the side of the bed.
13. Raise the side rail.
14. Raise the headrest to a sitting position.
15. Lower the side rail.
16. Slip one arm under the patient's neck and shoulders and support the neck and shoulder. Slip the other hand under the patient's far knee.
17. Turn the patient's body a quarter of a turn, letting the legs dangle over the edge of the mattress and holding the back upright.
18. Ask the patient to support some weight by pushing the fists into the mattress.
19. Help the patient adjust to this sitting position. Check pulse and respiration. Do not leave the patient unattended.
20. Help the patient put on the robe.
21. When the patient is to return to bed, reverse this procedure.
22. Lower the head of the bed, and help the patient move to the center of the bed.
23. Remove the slippers and the sheet.
24. Fold the top linens back over the patient and adjust them.
25. Raise the headrest to a safe and comfortable position.

26. Make sure the patient can reach the signal light.
27. Place the soiled sheet in the laundry bag, and return the robe and slippers to the closet.
28. Open the privacy curtain.
29. Wash your hands.

PROCEDURE: TURNING THE PATIENT ON THE SIDE FACING YOU

1. Wash your hands.
2. Check the patient's identification bracelet and speak the patient's name.
3. Explain that you are going to help the patient turn on the side.
4. Follow facility policy for asking visitors to leave the room.
5. Obtain three extra pillows.
6. Close the privacy curtain.
7. Lock the bed wheels, and raise the bed to a high level to ease your body movements.
8. Lower the headrest to the lowest level that is safe for the patient.
9. Stand on the side of the bed opposite to which the patient is to be turned.
10. Lower the near side rail, and make sure the far side rail is raised.
11. Move the patient to the side of the bed near you.
12. Cross the patient's arms over the chest.
13. Cross the patient's near leg over the far leg.
14. Raise the side rail.
15. Move the other side of the bed and lower the side rail.

16. Stand broadly with your feet 12 inches apart. Keeping your back straight, bend your knees.
17. Place one hand on the patient's far shoulder and the other hand on the patient's far hip.
18. Gently roll the patient's body toward you.
19. To support the patient's body, place one pillow against the back, and one under the patient's head and shoulder. Place a pillow in front of the bottom leg, bend the top leg, and place it on the pillow. Support the arm and hand with a pillow.
20. Raise the side rail.
21. Lower the bed to its lowest horizontal position.
22. Make sure the patient can reach the signal light.
23. Open the privacy curtain.
24. Wash your hands.

PROCEDURE: TURNING THE PATIENT ON THE SIDE FACING AWAY

1. Wash your hands.
2. Check the patient's identification bracelet and speak the patient's name.
3. Explain that you are going to help the patient turn on the side.
4. Follow facility policy for asking visitors to leave the room.
5. Obtain three extra pillows.
6. Close the privacy curtain.
7. Lock the bed wheels, and raise the bed to a high level to ease your body movements.
8. Lower the headrest to the lowest position safe for the patient.

9. Stand on the side of the bed away from which the patient will face.
10. Lower the near side rail, and make sure the far side rail is raised.
11. Loosen the top sheets without exposing the patient.
12. Move the patient to the side of the bed near you (see earlier procedure).
13. Cross the patient's arms over the chest; cross the patient's near leg over the far leg.
14. Stand broadly with your feet 12 inches apart. Keeping your back straight, bend your knees.
15. Hold the patient's near shoulder with one hand and the near hip with the other hand.
16. Gently push the patient's body away from you to the other side of the bed, rocking your body forward.
17. To support the patient's body, place one pillow against the back, and place another pillow under the patient's head and shoulder. Place a pillow in front of the bottom leg, bend the top leg, and place it on the pillow. Support the arm and hand with a pillow.
18. Adjust the top linens.
19. Raise the side rail.
20. Lower the bed to its lowest horizontal position.
21. Make sure the patient can reach the signal light.
22. Open the privacy curtain.
23. Wash your hands.

PROCEDURE: ROLLING THE PATIENT

1. Ask another nursing assistant to help you.
2. Wash your hands.

3. Check the patient's identification bracelet and speak the patient's name.
4. Explain that you are going to roll the patient on the side.
5. Follow facility policy for asking visitors to leave the room.
6. Obtain three extra pillows.
7. Close the privacy curtain.
8. Lock the bed wheels, and raise the bed to a high level to ease your body movements.
9 Lower the headrest to the lowest position safe for the patient.
10. Stand on the side of the bed away from which the patient will face.
11. Lower the near side rail, and make sure the far side rail is raised.
12. Move the patient to the side of the bed near you.
13. Cross the patient's arms on the chest, and place a pillow between the knees.
14. Raise the near side rail.
15. Move to the other side of the bed, and lower the side rail.
16. Stand near the patient's upper body, and ask your partner to stand near the patient's hips.
17. Stand broadly with your feet 12 inches apart.
18. Ask the patient to keep the whole body as rigid as possible.
19. Place one hand on the patient's near shoulder and one hand on the waist. Your partner should place one hand on the patient's hip and one hand on the legs.
20. At the same time, you and your partner should roll the patient toward you, making sure the patient is turned as a unit.

21. To support the patient's body, place a pillow against the back, and place a pillow under the head and neck. Adjust the pillow between the patient's legs, and support the arm and hand with a pillow.
22. Raise the side rail.
23. Lower the bed to its lowest horizontal position.
24. Make sure the patient can reach the signal light.
25. Open the privacy curtain.
26. Wash your hands.

General Rules for Transferring the Patient

- Always follow the principles of good body mechanics when transferring a patient (see earlier section).
- A partially helpless patient needs the help of at least one person in moving from the bed to a chair, wheelchair, or stretcher. Two or three people are necessary to help a helpless person move.
- Use a transfer belt when transferring a helpless patient from bed to chair or wheelchair and when helping the patient walk.
- When pushing a patient in a wheelchair, push from behind. Take precautions to avoid collisions at hallway intersections. To enter or exit an elevator, pull the wheelchair in or out after you.
- When transporting a patient on a stretcher, always use restraining straps; stay at the patient's head and push the stretcher feet first. Pull the stretcher into an elevator head first, and exit by pushing the stretcher out feet first.

■ To move down a ramp, take the wheelchair or stretcher down the ramp backward, facing the patient and walking backward.

PROCEDURE: USING A TRANSFER BELT

1. Wash your hands.
2. Check the patient's identification bracelet and speak the patient's name.
3. Explain that you are going to put a transfer belt on the patient.
4. Follow facility policy for asking visitors to leave the room.
5. Close the privacy curtain.
6. Lower the bed to its lowest horizontal position.
7. Help the patient sit up.
8. Put the transfer belt around the patient's waist over the clothing. Adjust the belt so that it has a snug and comfortable fit. Test this by putting your hand between the belt and body.
9. Shift the belt buckle so that it is off-center in the front or in the back.
10. Prepare to move the patient from the bed.

PROCEDURE: TRANSFERRING THE PATIENT FROM BED TO WHEELCHAIR

1. Wash your hands.
2. Check the patient's identification bracelet and speak the patient's name.
3. Explain that you are going to move the patient to a wheelchair.
4. Follow facility policy for asking visitors to leave the room.

5. Obtain a wheelchair, two bath blankets, patient's robe and slippers, a sheet, transfer belt (if necessary).
6. Close the privacy curtain.
7. If necessary, move furniture so that you and the patient can move easily.
8. Lock the bed wheels, and lower the bed to its lowest horizontal position.
9. Place the wheelchair at the head of the bed, with the back even with the headboard.
10. Fold a bath blanket and place it on the seat of the wheelchair. Lock the wheelchair wheels and raise the footrests.
11. Fold the top linens to the foot of the bed.
12. To protect the bottom linens, slip the sheet under the patient's feet.
13. Help the patient to sit on the side of the bed, making sure the feet touch the floor.
14. If necessary, put the transfer belt on the patient.
15. If you are using a transfer belt, help the patient stand up. Stand before the patient, and have the patient place hands on your shoulders. Bend your knees, bracing them against the patient's and blocking the patient's feet with yours. With both hands, grasp the transfer belt. Straighten your knees to pull the patient into a standing position.
16. If you are not using a transfer belt, stand before the patient and place your hands under the arms, holding the shoulder blades. Bend your knees, bracing them against the patient's knees and blocking the patient's feet with yours. On your count of three, have the patient push the fists into the mattress and

lean forward, and straighten your knees to pull the patient into a standing position.

17. Help the patient stand by holding the transfer belt or keeping your hands under the patient's arms. Support the patient's knees and feet with your knees and feet.

18. Help the patient turn and grasp first the far armrest of the wheelchair, then the near armrest.

19. Ask the patient to lean forward and bend the elbows and knees. Bending your knees, lower the patient into the wheelchair.

20. Help the patient position the buttocks against the back of the seat and assume a comfortable position.

21. Place the patient's feet on the footrests and adjust to a comfortable position.

22. Place a bath blanket on the patient's lap and legs, making sure the blanket cannot become caught in the wheels.

23. Remove the transfer belt if used.

24. Make sure the patient can reach the signal light.

25. Open the privacy curtain.

26. Wash your hands.

27. Report to the nurse that you have moved the patient to a wheelchair and how well the move was tolerated.

PROCEDURE: TRANSFERRING THE PATIENT FROM BED TO WHEELCHAIR WITH ASSISTANT

1. Ask another nursing assistant to help you.
2. Wash your hands.

3. Check the patient's identification bracelet and speak the patient's name.
4. Explain that you are going to move the patient to a wheelchair.
5. Follow facility policy for asking visitors to leave the room.
6. Obtain a wheelchair with removable armrests, two bath blankets, the patient's robe and slippers, and a pillow.
7. Close the privacy curtain.
8. If necessary, move furniture so that you and your partner can move easily.
9. Lock the wheels on the bed.
10. Place the wheelchair at the side of the bed, with the seat even with the patient's hips. Lock the wheels, and raise the footrests.
11. Fold a bath blanket and place it on the seat of the wheelchair.
12. Remove the armrest near the bed.
13. Fold the top linens to the foot of the bed.
14. Standing behind the wheelchair, slide your arms under the patient's arms and grasp the patient's forearms.
15. Ask your partner to stand in front of the wheelchair and grasp the patient's thighs and calves.
16. On your count of three, move the patient toward the wheelchair and into the seat.
17. Help the patient position the buttocks against the back of the seat and assume a comfortable position.
18. Replace the armrest.
19. Place the patient's feet on the footrests and adjust to a comfortable level.

20. Place a bath blanket on the patient's lap and legs, making sure the blanket cannot become caught in the wheelchair wheels.
21. Make sure the patient can reach the signal light.
22. Open the privacy curtain.
23. Wash your hands.
24. Report to the nurse that you have moved the patient to a wheelchair and how well the move was tolerated.

PROCEDURE: TRANSFERRING THE AMBULATORY PATIENT FROM WHEELCHAIR TO BED

1. Wash your hands.
2. Check the patient's identification bracelet and speak the patient's name.
3. Explain that you are going to help the patient get back into bed.
4. Follow facility policy for asking visitors to leave the room.
5. Close the privacy curtain.
6. Lock the bed wheels, and lower the bed to its lowest horizontal position.
7. Raise the headrest to a sitting position.
8. Place the wheelchair at the side of the bed, and lock the wheels.
9. Raise the footrests so that the patient's feet can touch the floor.
10. Unfasten the wheelchair's safety straps.
11. Lock arms with the patient.
12. At your count of three, have the patient lean forward, and help the patient stand, turn, and sit on the side of the bed.

13. Place one arm around the patient's shoulders and the other under the knees.
14. Keeping your back straight, bend your knees.
15. Slowly turn the patient's body, lifting the legs onto the mattress and lowering the shoulders against the headrest.
16. Lower the headrest.
17. Help the patient move to the center of the bed.
18. Place the pillow under the patient's head.
19. Adjust the top linens.
20. Raise the side rail.
21. Adjust the bed to a safe and comfortable position.
22. Make sure the patient can reach the signal light.
23. Open the privacy curtain.
24. Return the wheelchair to its proper location.
25. Wash your hands.
26. Report to the nurse that you have returned the patient to bed and how well the move was tolerated.

PROCEDURE: TRANSFERRING THE NONAMBULATORY PATIENT FROM WHEELCHAIR TO BED

1. Ask another nursing assistant for help.
2. Wash your hands.
3. Check the patient's identification bracelet and speak the patient's name.
4. Explain that you are going to move the patient back to bed.
5. Follow facility policy for asking visitors to leave the room.

6. Lock the bed wheels, and lower the bed to its lowest horizontal position.
7. Fold the top sheets to the foot of the bed.
8. Raise the headrest to a high sitting position.
9. Lower the near side rail.
10. Place the wheelchair at the side of the bed, and lock the wheels.
11. Raise the footrests and place the patient's feet on the floor.
12. Unfasten the wheelchair's safety straps.
13. With your partner, lock arms with the patient.
14. At your count of three, raise the patient's body, turn it, and sit the patient on the side of the bed.
15. Place the patient's head and shoulders against the headrest.
16. Ask your partner to support the patient's head and shoulders.
17. Gently lift the patient's legs onto the mattress.
18. Raise the side rail.
19. Lower the headrest.
20. Raise the bed to a high level to ease your body movements.
21. Move to the other side of the bed and lower that side rail.
22. Slip both arms under the patient's shoulders. Keeping your back straight and bending your knees, pull the shoulders toward you.
23. Slip both arms under the patient's buttocks. Keeping your back straight and bending your knees, pull the buttocks toward you.
24. Slip both arms under the patient's legs. Keeping your back straight and bending your knees, pull the legs toward you.

25. With the help of your partner, move the patient up in bed.
26. Place a pillow under the patient's head.
27. Adjust the top linens.
28. Lower the bed to a safe and comfortable position.
29. Raise the side rail.
30. Make sure the patient can reach the signal light.
31. Open the privacy curtain.
32. Return the wheelchair to its proper location.
33. Wash your hands.
34. Report to the nurse that you have returned the patient to bed and how well the move was tolerated.

PROCEDURE: MOVING THE PATIENT FROM BED TO STRETCHER

1. Ask one or two nursing assistants to help you.
2. Wash your hands.
3. Check the patient's identification bracelet and speak the patient's name.
4. Explain that you are going to move the patient onto a stretcher.
5. Follow facility policy for asking visitors to leave the room.
6. Obtain a stretcher, sheet or bath blanket, pillow.
7. Close the privacy curtain.
8. Raise the bed to the height of the stretcher, and lower the headrest to a flat position.
9. Lock the bed wheels.

10. Cover the patient with a bath blanket. Reaching under the blanket, fold the top linens to the foot of the bed. Loosen the drawsheet.
11. Lower the side rail on the side to which the patient will be moved.
12. With your partner, move the patient to the side of the bed, using the drawsheet.
13. Position the stretcher next to the bed, and lock the wheels. Ask your partner to stand on the other side of the bed.
14. Roll up the drawsheet to the patient's hips and torso.
15. Ask your partner to roll up the drawsheet on the other side of the patient's body.
16. Keeping your back straight, bend your knees, On your count of three, you and your partner should pull and slide the patient onto the stretcher.
17. Position the patient's body in the center of the stretcher. Support the head with a pillow if allowed.
18. Fasten the safety straps and raise the side rails.
19. Make sure the patient is covered with a blanket.
20. Wash your hands.
21. Report to the nurse that you have moved the patient to the stretcher and how well the move was tolerated.

PROCEDURE: MOVING THE PATIENT FROM STRETCHER TO BED

1. Ask one or two nursing assistants to help you.
2. Wash your hands.

3. Check the patient's identification bracelet and speak the patient's name.
4. Explain that you are going to move the patient to bed.
5. Follow facility policy for asking visitors to leave the room.
6. Lock the bed wheels.
7. Fold the top linens down to the foot of the bed.
8. Move the stretcher next to the bed, and lock the wheels.
9. Close the privacy curtain.
10. Raise the bed to the height of the stretcher, and lower the headrest to a flat position.
11. Ask your partner(s) to stand on the far side of the bed.
12. Lower the side rails.
13. Standing next to the stretcher, unfasten the safety straps.
14. Keeping your back straight, bend your knees.
15. On your count of three, you and your partner(s) should slide and pull the patient onto the bed. Use a pull sheet if possible.
16. Help the patient assume a comfortable position.
17. Reaching under the bath blanket, pull up the top linens. Remove the bath blanket and adjust the linens.
18. Lower the bed to a safe and comfortable position.
19. Raise the side rails.
20. Make sure the patient can reach the signal light.
21. Open the privacy curtain.
22. Wash your hands.

23. Report to the nurse that you have moved the patient from the stretcher to bed and how well the move was tolerated.

PROCEDURE: USING A MECHANICAL LIFT

1. Ask another nursing assistant for help.
2. Wash your hands.
3. Explain that you are going to move the patient with a mechanical lift.
4. Follow facility policy for asking visitors to leave the room.
5. Obtain a mechanical lift, a chair or wheelchair, a bath blanket, and the patient's slippers.
6. Close the privacy curtain.
7. Place the chair or wheelchair next to the bed, with the back even with the headboard. Place a folded bath blanket on the seat.
8. Lock the bed wheels, and lower the bed to its lowest level.
9. To position the sling, turn the patient from side to side and slide the sling under the body. The sling's lower edge should reach the patient's knees.
10. Raise the headrest to a sitting position.
11. Make sure the lift's release valve is in the closed position.
12. Widen the base of support by spreading the lift's legs. Lock the legs.
13. Holding the hooks as you move it, position the lift over the patient.
14. Ask the patient to fold both arms across the chest.

15. Attach the sling to the lift with the hooks. Be sure the short chain attaches to the back of the sling and the longer chain to the front of the sling. Be sure to keep the sharp edges of the hooks away from the patient's skin.
16. Attach the sling to the swivel bar.
17. Using the crank or pump, lift the patient off the bed.
18. Ask your partner to support the patient's legs.
19. Move the lift and patient away from the bed and toward the chair.
20. Lower the sling into the chair, and guide the patient's body to a sitting position.
21. Unhook the sling from the lift. Leave the sling under the patient.
22. Cover the patient with a bath blanket, making sure the blanket cannot become caught on the floor or in the wheelchair wheels.
23. Put the slippers on the patient's feet.
24. Fasten the wheelchair safety straps if necessary.
25. Make sure the patient can reach the signal light.
26. Open the privacy curtain.
27. Wash your hands.
28. Report to the nurse that you have moved the patient with a mechanical lift and how well the move was tolerated.
29. Reverse the procedure when the patient is to return to bed.

Chapter 7
Hygiene and Daily Care

This chapter includes information on the following:

*Procedure: Preventing bedsores in the
   incontinent patient*
Procedure: Caring for bedsores

Principles of Daily Care

▸ Early morning care to give (before breakfast):
  • Offer the bedpan or urinal
  • Help the patient with brushing teeth and oral
     hygiene
  • Help the patient wash hands and face
  • Give fresh drinking water
  • Arrange and straighten bed linens
  • Reposition patient if appropriate
▸ Morning care to give (after breakfast):
  • Offer the bedpan or urinal
  • Help the patient with brushing teeth and oral
     hygiene
  • Help the patient with a tub bath, shower, or
     bed bath
  • Help the patient change gowns or pajamas
  • Help the male patient shave his beard
  • Make the bed
  • Straighten the patient unit
▸ Afternoon care to give (after lunch and before
   visitors):
  • Offer the bedpan or urinal
  • Help the patient with brushing teeth and oral
     hygiene
  • Help the patient wash hands and face
  • Help patient brush or comb hair
  • Give fresh drinking water
  • Straighten the patient unit
▸ Evening care to give (after supper and before
   bedtime):
  • Offer the bedpan or urinal

- Help the patient with brushing teeth and oral hygiene
- Help the patient wash hands and face
- Give a backrub if appropriate
- Change soiled linen or gown
- Tighten bed linens

General Rules for Patient Hygiene Care

- Help the patient with hygiene care whenever needed--not just at scheduled times.
- For oral hygiene:
  - The nurse chooses what mouth care is needed for the patient
  - Report to the nurse cracked or blistered lips, bleeding, gums, or any mouth sores or white patches
  - Unconscious and NPO (nothing by mouth) patients receive oral hygiene every 2 hours to keep oral tissues moist
- For bathing the patient:
  - Decide with the nurse what kind of bath to give
  - Have all supplies and equipment ready before starting
  - Prevent falls
  - Maintain the patient's privacy
  - Prevent drafts in the room
  - Position yourself with good body mechanics
  - Carefully monitor the bath water temperature
  - Keep soap in the dish when not being handled
  - Rinse skin completely free of soap
  - Pat the skin dry instead of rubbing
  - Apply lubricant as appropriate

- Report to the nurse any redness, rashes, or broken skin
- For perineal care:
  - Patients who can should do their own perineal care
  - Be sensitive to the patient's likely embarrassment
  - Follow rules of asepsis: work from most clean to least clean areas
  - Use warm water, rinse thoroughly several times, and pat the area dry
- For giving a backrub:
  - Always check that it is safe to give the patient a backrub
  - Use warm lotion to reduce friction
  - Massage over all bony areas
  - Give the massage usually for 4 to 6 minutes

PROCEDURE: HELPING THE PATIENT BRUSH TEETH

1. Wash your hands.
2. Check the patient's identification bracelet and speak the patient's name.
3. Explain to the patient that you are going to help brush the teeth.
4. Follow facility policy for asking visitors to leave the room.
5. Collect the following equipment: toothbrush, toothpaste, mouthwash, dental floss, water cup, fresh water, straw, emesis basin, face towel.
6 Close the privacy curtain.

7. Raise the head of the bed to a comfortable sitting position.
8. Cover the patient's chest with the towel to protect the gown and bed linens.
9. Place all other equipment on the overbed table.
10. Lower the side rail.
11. Adjust the overbed table so that the patient can reach it.
12. Let the patient clean the teeth, helping if necessary.
13. Let the patient rinse the mouth with the water. Hold the emesis basin under the chin to enable the patient to spit out the rinse water.
14. When the patient is done, move the overbed table to the side of the bed and lower it to a comfortable position.
15. Adjust the head of the bed to a comfortable and safe level.
16. Raise the side rail.
17. Remove the soiled towel from the patient's chest.
18. Make sure the patient can reach the signal light.
19. Clean and return equipment to its proper place.
20. Discard any trash, and place soiled linens in the laundry bag.
21. Open the privacy curtain.
22. Wash your hands.
23. Report to the nurse any unusual observations, such as blisters, bleeding, swelling, irritation, or excessive redness in the mouth or on the lips and tongue.

PROCEDURE: BRUSHING THE PATIENT'S TEETH

1. Wash your hands.
2. Check the patient's identification bracelet and speak the patient's name.
3. Explain to the patient that you are going to clean the teeth.
4. Follow facility policy for asking visitors to leave the room.
5. Collect the following equipment: toothbrush, toothpaste, mouthwash, water cup, straw, emesis basin, towel, disposable gloves.
6. Close the privacy curtain.
7. Raise the bed to a high level to ease your body movements.
8. Raise the head of the bed to a comfortable sitting position. If the patient cannot sit up, position the patient on the side near you.
9. Cover the patient's chest with the towel to protect the gown and bed linens.
10. Place all other equipment on the overbed table.
11. Move the overbed table so that you can reach it easily.
12. Lower the side rail.
13. Put on the disposable gloves.
14. Pour water over the toothbrush, and apply toothpaste to it.
15. Clean the patient's teeth by positioning the brush horizontally against the outside surface of the teeth and brushing up and down on both sides and in front. Be sure to brush along the gumline. Then brush the inside surface of the front teeth by holding the brush

at a 45° angle and brushing with short strokes. To brush the inner surfaces of the remaining teeth, hold the brush horizontally against the teeth and brush back and forth. Then position the brush on top of the biting surfaces and brush back and forth. Brush the tongue gently.

16. Let the patient rinse with water, using the straw if necessary. Hold the emesis basin under the chin to allow the patient to spit out the rinse water.

17. Let the patient rinse with mouthwash, using the straw if necessary. Hold the emesis basin under the chin to allow the patient to spit out the mouthwash.

18. When the patient is done, move the overbed table to the side of the bed and lower it to a position comfortable for the patient.

19. Adjust the head of the bed to a comfortable and safe level.

20. Lower the bed to its lowest horizontal position.

21. Raise the side rail.

22. Remove the soiled towel from the patient's chest.

23. Make sure the patient can reach the signal light.

24. Clean and return equipment to its proper place.

25. Discard any trash and place soiled linens in the laundry bag.

26. Open the privacy curtain.

27. Wash your hands.

28. Report to the nurse any unusual observations, such as blisters, bleeding, swelling, irritation, or excessive redness in the mouth or on the lips or tongue.

PROCEDURE: FLOSSING THE PATIENT'S TEETH

1. Wash your hands.
2. Check the patient's identification bracelet and speak the patient's name.
3. Explain to the patient that you are going to floss the teeth.
4. Follow facility policy for asking visitors to leave the room.
5. Collect the following equipment: dental floss, emesis basin, water cup, water, straw, face towel, paper towels, disposable gloves.
6. Cover the overbed table with the paper towels, and place the remaining equipment on them.
7. Close the privacy curtain.
8. Raise the bed to a high level to ease your body movements.
9. Raise the head of the bed to a sitting position the patient finds comfortable. If the patient cannot sit up, position the patient on the side near you.
10. Cover the patient's chest with the towel to protect the gown and bed linens.
11. Move the overbed table so that you can reach it easily.
12. Lower the side rail.
13. Put on the disposable gloves.
14. Break off an 18-inch piece of dental floss.

15. To floss the upper teeth, wrap the floss ends on the middle fingers of each hand, and stretch the floss with your thumbs.
16. Begin with the upper back tooth on the right side, and clean the teeth by gently moving the floss up and down against each tooth. Be sure the floss reaches under the gumline. Floss each tooth in sequence, moving to the left side.
17. Adjust the floss to a new section after every two teeth.
18. To floss the lower teeth, hold the floss with your index fingers.
19. Begin with the lower back tooth on the right side, and clean the teeth by gently moving the floss up and down against each tooth. Be sure the floss reaches under the gumline. Floss each tooth in sequence, moving to the left side.
20. Let the patient rinse with water, using the straw if necessary. Hold the emesis basin under the chin to allow the patient to spit out the water.
21. When the patient is done, move the overbed table to the side of the bed and lower it to a position comfortable for the patient .
22. Adjust the head of the bed to a comfortable and safe level.
23. Lower the bed to its lowest horizontal position.
24. Raise the side rail.
25. Remove the soiled towel from the patient's chest.
26. Make sure the patient can reach the signal light.

27. Clean and return equipment to its proper place.
28. Discard any trash and place dirty linen in the laundry bag.
29. Open the privacy curtain.
30. Wash your hands.
31. Report to the nurse any unusual observations, such as blisters, bleeding, swelling, irritation, or excessive redness in the mouth or on the lips or tongue.

PROCEDURE: CARING FOR DENTURES

1. Wash your hands.
2. Check the patient's identification bracelet and speak the patient's name.
3. Explain to the patient that you are going to clean the dentures and how the patient can help.
4. Follow facility policy for asking visitors to leave the room.
5. Collect the following equipment: denture or toothbrush, denture cup identified with the patient's name and room number, denture cleaner or toothpaste, emesis basin, water cup, water, straw, mouthwash, two towels, gauze squares, disposable gloves.
6. Close the privacy curtain.
7. Cover the patient's chest with a towel to protect the gown and bed linens.
8. Raise the head of the bed to a comfortable sitting position. If the patient cannot sit up, position the patient on the side near you.
9. Lower the side rail.
10. Put on the disposable gloves.

11. If the patient can help, ask the patient to remove the dentures. Place them in the emesis basin.
12. If the patient cannot help, remove the dentures yourself. Using the gauze squares to touch the dentures, grasp the upper denture in one hand with your thumb and index fingers and remove from the mouth. If the denture is tightly in place, move it gently up and down, then remove it. Put the denture in the emesis basin. To remove the lower denture, grasp it in one hand with your thumb and index finger, move it slightly from left to right, and remove from the mouth. Put the denture in the emesis basin.
13. Raise the side rail.
14. Carry the emesis basin, denture cup, brush, and denture cleaner or toothpaste to the sink.
15. Using running water, rinse each denture and place it in the denture cup.
16. Place a clean towel on the bottom of the sink, and fill the sink half full with cool water.
17. Brush the dentures thoroughly, using horizontal strokes on the outer and biting surfaces and vertical strokes on the inner surfaces.
18. Return the dentures to the denture cup, and cover them with cool water.
19. Clean the emesis basin.
20. Place the denture cup and emesis basin on the bedside table.
21. Lower the side rail.

22. Let the patient rinse the mouth with mouthwash. Hold the emesis basin under the chin so the patient can spit out the mouthwash.
23. If the patient can help, ask the patient to insert the dentures.
24. If the patient cannot help, grasp the upper denture in one hand with your index finger and thumb. Raising the upper lip with your other hand, insert the denture into the patient's mouth. Using your index finger, press the denture securely into place. To insert the lower denture, grasp it in one hand with your index finger and thumb. Pull down the lower lip with your other hand, and place the denture into the patient's mouth. Using your index finger, gently push the denture into place.
25. If the patient is not going to wear the dentures, store them in a clean denture cup filled with cool water.
26. Adjust the head of the bed to a comfortable and safe level.
27. Lower the bed to its lowest horizontal position.
28. Raise the side rail.
29. Remove the soiled towel from the patient's chest.
30. Discard any trash and place dirty linen in the laundry bag.
31. Open the privacy curtain.
32. Wash your hands.
33. Report to the nurse any unusual observations, such as blisters, swelling, bleeding, irritation, or excessive redness in the mouth or on the lips or tongue.

PROCEDURE: MOUTH CARE FOR AN UNCONSCIOUS PATIENT

1. Wash your hands.
2. Check the patient's identification bracelet and speak the patient's name (who may still be able to hear you).
3. Explain to the patient that you are going to clean the mouth.
4. Follow facility policy for asking visitors to leave.
5. Collect the following equipment and place on bedside table: glycerine swabs, mouthwash, toothettes or other applicators, tongue depressor, water cup, water, towel, emesis basin, petroleum jelly, paper towels, disposable gloves.
6. Close the privacy curtain.
7. Raise the bed to a high level to ease your body movements, and lock the bed wheels in place.
8. Lower the side rail.
9. Put on the disposable gloves.
10. Position the patient's head to the side facing you.
11. Put the towel under the patient's face and neck.
12. Put the emesis basin under the patient's chin.
13. If the patient can respond, ask the patient to open the mouth. If the patient cannot respond, open the mouth by gently pressing the cheeks. Hold the tongue depressor on the tongue to separate the upper and lower teeth.

14. Clean the mouth with toothettes or applicators moistened with mouthwash. Wipe all tooth surfaces, the roof of the mouth, inner cheeks, lips, and tongue. Discard used applicators in the emesis basin.
15. Using applicators moistened with water, rinse all mouth surfaces in the same way.
16. Using the glycerine swabs, wipe all mouth surfaces. Do not overuse swabs, which can cause sores.
17. Apply petroleum jelly to the lips, following facility policy.
18. Remove the towel from beneath the patient's head and wipe the face.
19. Remove the disposable gloves.
20. Reposition the patient's head.
21. Adjust the head of the bed to a safe level.
22. Lower the bed to its lowest horizontal position.
23. Raise the side rail.
24. Discard any trash and place any dirty linens in the laundry bag.
25. Open the privacy curtain.
26. Wash your hands.
27. Report to the nurse any unusual observations, such as blisters, bleeding, swelling, irritation, or excessive redness in the mouth or on the lips or tongue.

PROCEDURE: HELPING THE PATIENT SHOWER

1. Wash your hands.
2. Check the patient's identification bracelet and speak the patient's name.

3. Explain that you are going to help the patient shower.
4. Follow facility policy for asking visitors to leave the room.
5. Collect the following equipment and place on a chair near the shower: rubber bath mat, disinfectant solution, two bath towels, floor mat, washcloth, soap, shower cap, clean gown.
6. To prepare the shower stall, wash the floor of the stall with disinfectant solution if necessary and place a rubber bath mat on the floor. Remove any electrical appliances from the stall. Place a floor mat outside the stall.
7. Close the privacy curtain.
8. Lower the side rail.
9. Help the patient sit on the side of the bed and put on robe and slippers.
10. Help the patient stand up and walk to the shower stall. If the patient has trouble walking, use a wheelchair or shower chair.
11. Show the patient the shower stall signal light and explain how to use it.
12. Turn on the water, adjusting the pressure and temperature to comfortable levels.
13. Help the patient to undress and into the shower. If the patient is using a shower chair, lock the wheels in place.
14. Hand the patient the soap and washcloth, helping the patient bathe if necessary.
15. Open a towel on the chair outside the stall.
16. When the patient signals being done, turn off the water.
17. Help the patient out of the stall and sit on the towel-covered chair.

18. Help the patient dry off by patting gently with a towel.
19. Help the patient to put on the clean gown, robe, and slippers.
20. Walk the patient back to the room and to bed.
21. Raise the side rails.
22. Adjust the head of the bed to a safe and comfortable level.
23. Open the privacy curtain.
24. Return to the shower stall, and remove all soiled linen and place in the laundry bag. Discard any trash.
25. Wash your hands.
26. Report to the nurse how well the patient tolerated the shower and any unusual observations, such as skin irritation or sores.

PROCEDURE: HELPING THE PATIENT WITH A TUB BATH

1. Wash your hands.
2. Check the patient's identification bracelet and speak the patient's name.
3. Explain that you are going to help the patient take a tub bath.
4. Follow facility policy for asking visitors to leave the room.
5. Collect the following equipment and place it on a chair near the tub: rubber bath mat, disinfectant solution, washcloth, two bath towels, floor mat, soap, bath thermometer, clean gown.

6. To prepare the bath tub, wash it with disinfectant solution and place a rubber bath mat on the bottom. Remove any electrical appliances from the tub. Place a floor mat in front of the tub.
7. Close the privacy curtain.
8. Lower the side rail.
9. Help the patient sit on the side of the bed and put on robe and slippers.
10. Help the patient stand up and walk to the bath tub. If the patient has trouble walking, help with a wheelchair.
11. Help the patient sit on the chair next to the tub.
12. Show the patient the bath tub signal light and how to use it.
13. Fill the tub halfway with 105° F (40.5° C) water, testing the temperature with the bath thermometer.
14. Help the patient to undress and to climb into the tub.
15. Hand the patient the soap and washcloth, helping bathe if necessary.
16. Let the patient stay in the tub no longer than your instructions permit.
17. Open a towel on the chair near the tub.
18. When done, help the patient climb out of the tub and sit on the towel-covered chair.
19. Help the patient dry off by patting gently with a towel.
20. Help the patient to put on the clean gown, robe, and slippers.
21. Help the patient walk back to the room and to bed.
22. Raise the side rails.

23. Adjust the head of the bed to a safe and comfortable level.
24. Open the privacy curtain.
25. Return to the bath tub, and remove all soiled linen and place in the laundry bag. Discard any trash.
26. Wash your hands.
27. Report to the nurse how well the patient tolerated the bath and any unusual observations, such as skin irritation or sores.

PROCEDURE: GIVING A BED BATH

1. Wash your hands.
2. Check the patient's identification bracelet and speak the patient's name.
3. Explain to the patient that you are going to give a bed bath and how to help.
4. Follow facility policy for asking visitors to leave the room.
5. Collect the following equipment: wash basin, soap and soap dish, washcloth, bath thermometer, orange stick, bath towels, face towels, bath blanket, clean gown, body lotion, equipment for cleaning the mouth, brush and comb, disposable gloves, paper towels.
6. Close the privacy curtain.
7. Offer the patient the bedpan or urinal.
8. Raise the bed to a high level to ease your body movements.
9. Remove the signal light.
10. Put on the disposable gloves.
11. Help the patient to clean the mouth and teeth.

12. Remove top linens, taking care not to expose the patient. Place the bath blanket over the patient.
13. Lower the bed's headrest and kneerest to a flat position that is comfortable and safe for the patient.
14. Cover the overbed table with paper towels.
15. Fill the wash basin two-thirds full with 115° F (46° C) water, testing the temperature with the bath thermometer.
16. Place the wash basin on the overbed table.
17. Lower the side rail.
18. Help the patient move to the side of the bed closest to you.
19. Cover the patient's chest with a face towel.
20. To wash the patient's face, make a mitt with the washcloth and rinse it in water only. Wash the patient's eyes from the inner corner to the outside. Ask the patient about having the face washed with soap. Wash the face, ears, and neck. Rinse and pat dry gently with the towel on the patient's chest.
21. Remove the patient's gown, keeping the body covered with the bath blanket. If the patient is wearing jewelry, remove it and place in the drawer of the bedside table.
22. Place a bath towel lengthwise under the patient's arm farthest from you. Support the arm with the palm of your hand under the patient's elbow. Wash the shoulder, armpit, and arm, using long, circular strokes. Rinse and pat dry.
23. Place the wash basin on the towel, and put the patient's hand into the water. Wash the hand. Clean gently under the fingernails with

the orange stick. Rinse and pat the hand dry.
Remove the wash basin and cover the hand
with the bath blanket.

24. Clean the patient's other arm, shoulder,
    armpit, and hand in the same way.

25. Place a bath towel across the patient's chest.
    Holding the towel in place, slide the bath
    blanket down to the patient's abdomen. Wash
    the patient's chest. Rinse and pat dry.

26. Move the towel so that it covers the patient's
    chest and abdomen lengthwise, taking care
    not to expose the patient. Slide the bath
    blanket down to the pubic area. Wash the
    patient's abdomen. Rinse and pat dry. Pull
    the bath blanket to cover the abdomen and
    chest, and remove the towel.

27. If the water is dirty or cool, empty the wash
    basin and refill it with clean 115° F (46° C)
    water. Be sure to raise the side rail before
    leaving the bed.

28. Unfold the bath blanket to expose the leg
    farthest from you, taking care not to expose
    the genital area. Put a bath towel lengthwise
    under the leg and foot.

29. Bend the knee and hold the leg with one arm.
    Wash the leg with long strokes. Rinse and pat
    dry.

30. Place the wash basin on the towel. If the
    patient can help, ask the patient to bend the
    knee and put the foot in the wash basin. If the
    patient cannot help, lift the leg off the mattress
    and slide the basin under the foot.

31. Wash the foot. Use the orange stick to clean
    gently under the toenails. Rinse and remove
    the foot from the basin. Pat it dry. Cover the

leg and foot with the bath blanket and remove the towel.

32. Clean the patient's other leg and foot in the same way.
33. Empty the wash basin and refill it with clean 115° F (46° C) water. Be sure to raise the side rail before leaving the bed.
34. Help the patient to turn on the side with back toward you, making sure the body remains covered with the bath blanket.
35. Place a bath towel lengthwise against the patient's back. Wash the back and neck, using long, circular strokes. Rinse and pat dry. Give the patient a back massage, using lubricant, especially over bony areas. Remove the towel.
36. Help the patient turn onto the back.
37. If the patient can help, ask the patient to wash the genital area. Provide a clean, soapy washcloth, a clean wet washcloth for rinsing, and a dry towel. If the patient cannot do this, wash and dry the genital area yourself, making sure you do not expose it.
38. Help the patient put on a clean gown.
39. Comb and brush the patient's hair.
40. Return the jewelry if the patient wants it.
41. Make the bed and attach the signal light within the patient's reach.
42. Raise the side rails.
43. Lower the bed to its lowest horizontal position.
44. Raise the headrest to a comfortable and safe level.

45. Clean and return the equipment to its proper place. Wipe off the overbed table with the paper towels. Put soiled linens in the laundry bag, and discard any trash.
46. Open the privacy curtain.
47. Wash your hands.
48. Report to the nurse how well the patient tolerated the bath and any unusual observations, such as skin irritation or sores.

PROCEDURE: GIVING A PARTIAL BED BATH

1. Wash your hands.
2. Check the patient's identification bracelet and speak the patient's name.
3. Explain that you are going to help the patient take a partial bed bath.
4. Follow facility policy for asking visitors to leave the room.
5. Collect the following equipment: equipment for cleaning the mouth, wash basin, soap and soap dish, washcloth, bath thermometer, bath and face towels, clean gown, bath blanket, orange stick, body lotion, comb and hair brush, paper towels, disposable gloves. Collect clean bed linens and place on the bedside chair.
6. Close the privacy curtain.
7. Offer the patient the bedpan or urinal.
8. Raise the bed to a high level to ease your body movements.
9. Put on the disposable gloves.
10. Help the patient to clean the mouth and teeth.

11. Remove top linens, taking care not to expose the patient. Place the bath blanket over the patient.
12. Cover the overbed table with paper towels.
13. Fill the wash basin two-thirds full with 115° F (46° C) water, testing the temperature with the bath thermometer.
14. Place the wash basin on the overbed table.
15. Raise the head of the bed to a comfortable sitting position.
16. Help the patient remove the gown, keeping the body covered with the bath blanket. If the patient is wearing jewelry, help remove it and place it in the drawer of the bedside table.
17. Place the overbed table so that the patient can reach the wash basin easily. Be sure the signal light is within the patient's reach.
18. Ask the patient to wash the parts of the body that the patient can reach easily. Explain that you will help wash inaccessible areas such as the back. Ask the patient to signal you when done.
19. Wash your hands and leave the room.
20. When the patient signals you, knock and enter the room.
21. Wash your hands and put on the disposable gloves.
22. Empty the wash basin and refill it with clean 115° F (46° C) water.
23. Wash the areas the patient could not reach, following the procedures for a complete bed bath.
24. Give the patient a back massage.

25. Help the patient put on a clean gown, taking care not to expose him. Return the jewelry if the patient wants it.
26. Help the patient comb and brush the hair.
27. If allowed out of bed, help the patient to the bedside chair. If the patient cannot leave the bed, help the patient turn to the side away from you.
28. Make the bed and attach the signal light within the patient's reach.
29. Lower the bed to its lowest horizontal position.
30. If the patient is out of bed, help the patient to return to bed.
31. Raise the side rails.
32. Raise the headrest to a comfortable and safe position.
33. Clean and return the equipment to its proper place. Wipe off the overbed table with the paper towels. Place soiled linens in the laundry bag, and discard any trash.
34. Open the privacy curtain.
35. Wash your hands.
36. Report to the nurse how well the patient tolerated the bath and any unusual observations, such as skin irritation or sores.

PROCEDURE: COMBING THE PATIENT'S HAIR

1. Wash your hands.
2. Check the patient's identification bracelet and speak the patient's name.
3. Explain to the patient that you are going to comb the hair.
4. Follow facility policy for asking visitors to leave the room.

5. Collect the following equipment and place on the bedside table: comb and brush, bath towel.
6. Close the privacy curtain.
7. Lower the side rail.
8. Raise the bed's headrest to a comfortable sitting position, and help the patient to sit up.
9. If the patient is sitting up, cover the shoulders with the towel. If patient cannot sit up, place the towel on the pillow under the head.
10. If the patient wears glasses, ask for them to be removed. Put the glasses in their case, if available, and store in the bedside table drawer.
11. Carefully comb or brush small sections of hair, starting at the hair ends and moving in to the scalp.
12. Style the hair as the patient wishes.
13. Remove the towel.
14. Return the eyeglasses, if any, to the patient.
15. Raise the side rail.
16. Adjust the headrest to a comfortable and safe position.
17. Make sure the patient can reach the signal light.
18. Open the privacy curtain.
19. Clean and return equipment to its proper place, and place soiled linens in the laundry bag. Discard any trash.
20. Wash your hands.
21. Report to the nurse that you have combed the patient's hair and any unusual observations.

PROCEDURE: WASHING THE PATIENT'S HAIR

1. Wash your hands.
2. Check the patient's identification bracelet and speak the patient's name.
3. Explain to the patient that you are going to shampoo the hair and how to help.
4. Follow facility policy for asking visitors to leave the room.
5. Collect the following equipment and place on the bedside table: shampoo, bath towels, washcloth, bath thermometer, water trough, two water basins, bath blanket, waterproof bed protector, comb and brush, hair dryer, paper cup, cotton.
6. Close the privacy curtain.
7. Raise the bed to its highest horizontal position.
8. Gently insert small pieces of cotton into the patient's ears to keep them dry.
9. Comb and brush smooth the patient's hair.
10. Place the bedside chair next to bed, with the back touching the mattress.
11. Put one basin on the chair.
12. Help the patient to move to the side of the bed near the chair.
13. Remove the pillow and insert it under the small of the patient's back.
14. Cover the patient with the bath blanket. Taking care not to expose the patient, reach under the bath blanket and pull the top linens down to the patient's abdomen.
15. Place the waterproof bed protector under the patient's head.

16. Place the water trough under the patient's head, making sure the water outlet is directed toward the basin at the side of the bed.
17. Fill the other basin with clean water at 110° F (43° C) or the temperature used in your facility, testing the temperature with the bath thermometer.   Place the basin on the bedside table.
18. Place the washcloth over the face and ask the patient to hold it there.
19. Fill the paper cup with water and wet the patient's hair thoroughly.
20. Using a small amount of shampoo, wash the patient's hair, starting at the hair line and moving to the back of the head. Massage the scalp by pressing firmly with your fingers.
21. Rinse the hair with clean water, making sure all shampoo is removed.
22. Using the washcloth, dry the patient's face.
23. Remove the cotton from the patient's ears.
24. Wrap the patient's head in a bath towel, rubbing the hair and scalp gently.
25. Remove the water trough and waterproof bed protector. Reaching under the bath blanket, pull up the top linens and straighten them. Remove the bath blanket. Remove the pillow from under the patient's back and place it under the patient's head.
26. Comb the patient's hair to remove tangles.
27. Dry the hair with the hair dryer.
28. Lower the bed and adjust the backrest to a comfortable and safe position.
29. Clean and return all equipment to the proper place. Place soiled linens in the laundry bag, and discard any trash.

30. Make sure the patient can reach the signal light.
31. Wash your hands.
32. Report to the nurse that you have shampooed the patient's hair and any unusual observations.

PROCEDURE: SHAVING THE PATIENT'S BEARD

1. Wash your hands.
2. Check the patient's identification bracelet and speak his name.
3. Explain to the patient that you are going to shave his beard and how he can help.
4. Follow facility policy for asking visitors to leave the room.
5. Collect the following equipment and place on the bedside table: washcloth, bath towel, water basin, bath thermometer, shaving cream, shaving brush, safety razor, tissues, aftershave lotion.
6. Close the privacy curtain.
7. Raise the bed to a high level to ease your body movements.
8. Fill the water basin with 115° F (46° C) water, testing the temperature with the bath thermometer. Place on the bedside table.
9. Lower the side rail.
10. If allowed, raise the backrest so that the patient is sitting partially upright.
11. Adjust the light to shine on the patient's face.
12. Cover the patient's chest and shoulders with the bath towel.

13. Wet the washcloth and wring it out. Pat the patient's face with the damp wash cloth to soften the beard.
14. Using the shaving brush, apply a generous amount of shaving cream to the beard.
15. Holding the skin taut with one hand, shave in the direction of hair growth. Start near the ears, work downward over the cheeks, then use shorter strokes on the chin and lips. Stroke upward on the neck under the chin. Rinse the razor frequently.
16. If the skin is nicked, apply direct pressure with a damp tissue.
17. Using the washcloth, wash off any remaining shaving cream. Dry the face with the bath towel.
18. If the patient wishes, apply aftershave lotion.
19. Lower the bed and adjust the backrest to a safe and comfortable position.
20. Raise the side rail.
21. Clean and return all equipment to its proper place, and place soiled linens in the laundry bag. Discard any trash.
22. Make sure the patient can reach the signal light.
23. Open the privacy curtain.
24. Wash your hands.
25. Report to the nurse that you have shaved the patient and any unusual observations, including nicks or bleeding.

PROCEDURE: CARING FOR THE PATIENT'S NAILS AND FEET

1. Wash your hands.

2. Check the patient's identification bracelet and speak the patient's name.
3. Explain to the patient that you are going to clean the nails and feet.
4. Follow facility policy for asking visitors to leave the room.
5. Collect the following equipment and place on the overbed table: wash basin, bath thermometer, emesis basin, nail clippers, orange stick, nail file or emery board, lotion, paper towels, bath mat, bath towel, face towel, washcloth, hand lotion, bed protector (if necessary).
6. Close the privacy curtain.
7. If the patient cannot leave the bed, raise the bed to a high level to ease your body movements. Raise the bed's headrest to a comfortable and safe sitting position. Position the bed protector under the patient's feet, then cover it with a bath towel.
8. If the patient can leave the bed, lower the side rail. Then help the patient sit on the side of the bed and put on the robe. Help the patient stand up and walk to the bedside chair. Be sure the patient can reach the signal light. Put the bathmat on the floor under the patient's feet.
9. Fill the wash basin halfway with water at 110° F (43° C) or at the temperature used in your facility, testing the temperature with the bath thermometer.
10. Place the wash basin under the patient's feet, and help the patient put the feet into the basin.

11. Move the overbed table so that the patient can reach it easily.
12. Fill the emesis basin halfway with water at 110° F (43° C) or at the temperature used in your facility, testing the temperature with the bath thermometer.
13. Cover the overbed table with paper towels, and place the emesis basin on the towels.
14. Place the patient's fingers into the emesis basin for soaking.
15. Ask the patient to let the fingers and feet soak for at least 20 minutes. Check the water temperature after 10 minutes, and change the water if it is cool.
16. Remove the emesis basin and dry the fingers.
17. Using the orange stick, clean under the fingernails and push the cuticles back gently.
18. If the nails are long, clip them with the nail clippers.
19. Smooth nail ends with a nail file or emery board.
20. Rub the hands with lotion.
21. Remove the overbed table.
22. Remove the wash basin and dry the patient's feet.
23. Use the same procedure to clean the patient's toenails.
24. Using a wet washcloth, rub any callused areas on the feet. Dry the patient's feet.
25. Rub the feet and ankles with lotion.
26. If the patient is in bed, remove the bed protector and towel.
27. If the patient is in the chair, help the patient remove the robe and walk back to bed.
28. Raise the side rails.

29. Adjust the head of the bed to a safe and comfortable level.
30. Open the privacy curtain.
31. Make sure the signal light is within the patient's reach.
32. Clean and return equipment to its proper place, and place all soiled linen in the laundry bag. Discard any trash.
33. Wash your hands.
34. Report to the nurse that you cleaned the patient's nails and feet and any unusual observations, such as skin irritation or callused areas.

PROCEDURE: MALE PERINEAL CARE

1. Wash your hands.
2. Check the patient's identification bracelet and speak his name.
3. Follow facility policy for asking visitors to leave the room.
4. Explain to the patient that you are going to clean his genital area and how he can help.
5. Collect the following equipment and place on the bedside table: wash basin, bath thermometer, soap and soap dish, disposable washcloths, bath towel, bath blanket, waterproof bed protector, disposable gloves, paper towels.
6. Close the privacy curtain.
7. Raise the bed to a high level to ease your body movements.
8. Lower the side rail.
9. Place the bath blanket over the patient.

10. Reaching under the bath blanket, pull the top linens down to the foot of the bed, taking care not to expose the patient.
11. Place the waterproof bed protector under the patient's buttocks.
12. To ensure privacy, drape the bath blanket diagonally across the patient, so that one corner is at his neck and another is between his legs. Wrap the other two corners once around the patient's legs and tuck under each hip.
13. Raise the side rail.
14. Fill the wash basin with 105° F (41° C) water, testing the temperature with the bath thermometer.
15. Cover the overbed table with paper towels, and place the wash basin on the towels.
16. Lower the side rail.
17. Put on the disposable gloves.
18. Help the patient spread his legs apart and flex his knees.
19. Fold the corner of the bath blanket that is between the patient's legs up onto his abdomen.
20. Place the disposable washcloths in the wash basin. Squeezing out the water, apply soap to one.
21. Holding the penis, wash gently with the washcloth. Start at the tip and move outward, then clean the shaft. If the patient is uncircumcised, pull back the foreskin. Rinse the penis with a fresh washcloth and return the foreskin, if any, to its natural position.
22. Using a new soapy washcloth, clean the scrotum and rinse well.

23. Dry the penis and scrotum with a towel.
24. Fold the corner of the bath blanket back between the patient's legs.
25. Help the patient lower his knees and turn onto his side facing away from you.
26. Using a new soapy washcloth, clean the rectal area by wiping from the scrotal area back to the anus. Use only one stroke. Repeat with fresh washcloths until the area is clean.
27. Rinse the rectal area using the same wiping motion. Repeat with fresh washcloths until the area is rinsed.
28. Dry the rectal area with a towel.
29. Remove the waterproof bed protector.
30. Remove the disposable gloves and discard them.
31. Help the patient turn onto his back.
32. Reaching under the bath blanket, return top linens to their proper position. Remove the bath blanket.
33. Raise the side rail.
34. Lower the bed to its lowest horizontal position.
35. Adjust the head of the bed to a safe and comfortable position.
36. Wipe the overbed table with the paper towels.
37. Clean and return equipment to its proper location. Place soiled linens in the laundry bag, and discard any trash.
38. Make sure the patient can reach the signal light.
39. Open the privacy curtain.
40. Wash your hands.
41. Report to the nurse that you have cleaned the patient's perineal area and any unusual observations, such as sores, irritation,

swelling, or discharge, or any patient
complaints, such as burning or pain.

PROCEDURE: FEMALE PERINEAL CARE

1. Wash your hands.
2. Check the patient's identification bracelet and
    speak her name.
3. Follow facility policy for asking visitors to leave
    the room.
4. Explain to the patient that you are going to
    clean her genital area and how she can help.
5. Collect the following equipment and place on
    the bedside table: Wash basin, bath
    thermometer, soap and soap dish, disposable
    washcloths, bath towel, bath blanket,
    waterproof bed protector, disposable gloves,
    paper towels.
6. Close the privacy curtain.
7. Raise the bed to a high level to ease your
    body movements.
8. Lower the side rail.
9. Place the bath blanket over the patient.
10. Reaching under the bath blanket, pull the top
    linens down to the foot of the bed, taking care
    not to expose the patient.
11. Place the waterproof bed protector under the
    patient's buttocks.
12. To ensure privacy, drape the bath blanket
    diagonally across the patient, so that one
    corner is at her neck and another is between
    her legs. Wrap the other two corners once
    around the patient's legs and tuck under each
    hip.
13. Raise the side rail.

14. Fill the wash basin with 105° F (41° C) water, testing the temperature with the bath thermometer.
15. Cover the overbed table with paper towels, and place the wash basin on the towels.
16. Lower the side rail.
17. Put on the disposable gloves.
18. Help the patient spread her legs apart and flex her knees.
19. Fold the corner of the bath blanket that is between the patient's legs up onto her abdomen.
20. Place the disposable washcloths in the wash basin. Squeezing out the water, apply soap to one.
21. Wash the genitals by separating the labia (folds) with one hand and wiping, front to back, with the washcloth held in the other hand. Be sure to wipe only once with each washcloth. Repeat with fresh washcloths until the area is clean. (If disposable washcloths are not available, use a cloth and turn it to clean with the other side.)
22. Rinse the genitals using the same motion. Repeat with fresh washcloths until the area is rinsed.
23. Dry the genital area with a towel.
24. Fold the corner of the bath blanket back between the patient's legs.
25. Help the patient lower her knees, and help her turn onto her side facing away from you.
26. Using a new soapy washcloth, clean the rectal area by wiping from the vaginal area back to the anus. Use only one stroke. Repeat with fresh washcloths until the area is clean.

27. Rinse the rectal area using the same wiping motion. Repeat with fresh washcloths until the area is rinsed.
28. Dry the rectal area with a towel.
29. Remove the waterproof bed protector.
30. Remove the disposable gloves and discard them.
31. Help the patient turn onto her back.
32. Reaching under the bath blanket, return top linens to their proper position. Remove the bath blanket.
33. Raise the side rail.
34. Lower the bed to its lowest horizontal position.
35. Adjust the head of the bed to a safe and comfortable position.
36. Wipe the overbed table with the paper towels.
37. Clean and return equipment to its proper place. Put the soiled linens in the laundry bag, and discard any trash.
38. Make sure the patient can reach the signal light.
39. Open the privacy curtain.
40. Wash your hands.
41. Report to the nurse that you have cleaned the patient's perineal area and any unusual observations, such as sores, irritation, swelling, or discharge, or any patient complaints, such as burning or pain.

PROCEDURE: PERFORMING A VAGINAL IRRIGATION

1. Wash your hands.
2. Check the patient's identification bracelet and speak her name.

3. Follow facility policy for asking visitors to leave the room.
4. Explain to the patient that you are going to give her a vaginal irrigation (douche) and how she can help.
5. Collect the following equipment: bedpan and cover, bath blanket, disposable douche kit (container, tubing, clamp, and nozzle), irrigation solution, toilet tissue, waterproof bed protector, disposable gloves, equipment for perineal care.
6. Close the privacy curtain and the door.
7. Raise the bed to a high level to ease your body movements.
8. Give the patient the bedpan and toilet tissue, and ask her to empty her bladder to ensure the procedure's success.
9. When the patient is done, remove the bedpan. If required, measure and record output on the appropriate form. Empty and clean the bedpan and place it on the bedside chair.
10. Wash your hands.
11. Lower the side rail.
12. Place the bath blanket over the patient.
13. Reaching under the bath blanket, pull the top linens down to the foot of the bed, taking care not to expose the patient.
14. Place the waterproof bed protector under the patient's buttocks.
15. To ensure privacy, drape the bath blanket diagonally across the patient, so that one corner is at her neck and another is between her legs. Wrap the other two corners once around the patient's legs and tuck under each hip.

16. Wash your hands and put on disposable gloves.
17. Provide perineal care.
18. Help the patient position herself on the bedpan, spread her legs apart, and flex her knees.
19. Open the douche kit and clamp closed the irrigation tubing.
20. Pour the irrigation solution into the irrigation container.
21. Place the irrigation container on the IV pole, allowing the container to hang about 12 inches above the patient's vagina.
22. Place the nozzle over the patient's genital area. Unclamp the tubing to expel any air and to moisten the genital area with some solution.
23. Gently insert the nozzle tip 3 inches into the patient's vagina.
24. Rotating the nozzle slowly, allow the solution to flow into the vagina.
25. When the solution has completely drained from the container, clamp the tubing closed.
26. Gently remove the nozzle from the vagina. Put the tubing into the irrigation container.
27. Help the patient to sit up on the bedpan, so that the solution can drain from the vagina. If permitted, raise the back of the bed to increase the patient's comfort.
28. Using toilet tissue, thoroughly dry the perineal area. Discard the tissue into the bedpan.
29. Remove the bedpan and the bed protector.
30. Lower the bed to its lowest horizontal position.
31. Reaching under the bath blanket, return top linens to their proper position. Remove the bath blanket.

32. Change linen if damp.
33. Raise the side rail.
34. Adjust the head of the bed to a safe and comfortable position.
35. Inspect the contents of the bedpan. If the returned solution is unclear or discolored, collect a sample. Empty and wash the bedpan.
36. Clean and return equipment to its proper place. Put soiled linens in the laundry bag, and discard any trash.
37. Make sure the patient can reach the signal light.
38. Open the privacy curtain and door.
39. Wash your hands.
40. Report to the nurse that you have performed a vaginal irrigation, any usual observations, such as genital irritations or sores, and whether you collected a sample of returned solution.

PROCEDURE: CHANGING THE PATIENT'S GOWN

1. Wash your hands.
2. Check the patient's identification bracelet and speak the patient's name.
3. Follow facility policy for asking visitors to leave the room.
4. Explain to the patient that you are going to change the gown.
5. Obtain a clean gown.
6. Raise the bed to a high level to ease your body movements.
7. Lower the side rail.

8. Help the patient turn on the side facing away from you. Untie the gown. If the patient cannot move, reach under the neck and untie the gown.

9. Pull the gown loose around the patient's body. Cover the patient with the top sheets.

10. Unfold the clean gown, and place it on the patient's chest.

11. Remove each sleeve of the old gown from the patient's arms. If the patient has an injured arm, remove the sleeve from the unaffected arm first. Then, supporting the injured arm in one hand, grasp the sleeve in the other hand and slip it up the patient's wrist and arm.

12. Slide each arm through the sleeve of the clean gown. If the patient has an injured arm, slip the sleeve on the injured arm first, then slide the unaffected arm through the other sleeve.

13. Reaching under the top sheets, remove the old gown.

14. Tie the new gown. If the patient prefers, tie the gown only at the neck so that the patient will not lie on knots.

15. Lower the bed to a safe and comfortable position.

16. Raise the side rail.

17. Make sure the patient can reach the signal light.

18. Place the soiled gown in the laundry bag.

19. Wash your hands.

20. Report to the nurse that you have changed the patient's gown and any unusual observations.

PROCEDURE: DRESSING A PATIENT IN STREET CLOTHES

1. Wash your hands.
2. Check the patient's identification bracelet and speak the patient's name.
3. Explain that you are going to help the patient dress.
4. Follow facility policy for asking visitors to leave the room.
5. Collect the patient's clothing and a bath blanket.
6. Close the privacy curtain and the door.
7. Raise the bed to a high level to ease your body movements.
8. Lower the side rail.
9. Help the patient to lie on the back. Cover the patient with the bath blanket, and fold the top linens down to the foot of the bed.
10. Undress the patient if necessary, taking care not to expose the body.
11. Dress the patient using the following movements, starting with underclothing and finishing with sock and shoes.
12. For clothes that are pulled over the head, first slip the neck of the garment over the patient's head. Starting with the patient's weaker side, raise the arm gently and slip the arm and shoulders into the garment. Then repeat with the patient's stronger side. Pull the garment down to the patient's waist.
13. For clothes that open in front, first slide the garment onto the patient's weaker arm and shoulder. Locking arms with the patient, lift the head and shoulders enough to pull the

garment around to the other side. Lower the
patient, and slide the garment onto the other
arm and shoulder. Close buttons, snaps, or
zippers.

14. For slacks and pants, put both feet into the
    pants and slide up the patient's legs to the
    hips. If the patient can help, ask the patient to
    lift the hips off the bed. Pull the pants up over
    the hips, and ask the patient to ease back
    onto the bed. If the patient cannot do this,
    help turn the patient onto the stronger side.
    Slip the pants over the weaker hip, then help
    the patient to turn onto the weaker side. Slip
    the pants onto the strong hip, then button or
    zip the pants. If the patient is wearing a
    catheter, pin the pants closed. Help the
    patient resume the original position.

15. For clothes that open in the back, first slip the
    garment onto the patient's weaker arm and
    shoulder, then slip it onto the other arm and
    shoulder. Locking arms with the patient, lift
    the head and shoulders enough to pull the
    garment around to the back. Close buttons,
    snaps, or zippers.

16. To put on socks or stockings, roll the sock
    down from the opening to the heel. Slip the
    sock over the toes and pull past the heel and
    up the leg.

17. To put on shoes, loosen any laces first and,
    supporting the patient's ankle, slide the toes,
    foot, and heel into the shoe.

18. Remove the bath blanket. Help the patient out
    of bed and into the chair. If the patient cannot
    leave the bed, put the bed in its lowest

horizontal position and adjust the top linens.
Raise the side rail.
19. Make sure the patient can reach the signal
light.
20. Open the privacy curtain and the door.
21. Place soiled gown and linens in the laundry
bag.
22. Wash your hands.
23. Report to the nurse that you have dressed the
patient and any unusual observations.

PROCEDURE: UNDRESSING A PATIENT IN STREET CLOTHES

1. Wash your hands.
2. Check the patient's identification bracelet and
speak the patient's name.
3. Explain that you are going to help the patient
undress.
4. Follow facility policy for asking visitors to leave
the room.
5. Collect a bath blanket and a gown or the
patient's clothing.
6. Close the privacy curtain.
7. Raise the bed to a high level to ease your
body movements.
8. Lower the side rail.
9. Cover the patient with the bath blanket.
Reaching under the bath blanket, pull the top
linens down to the foot of the bed, taking care
not to expose the patient.
10. To remove the patient's shoes, loosen
shoelaces or buckles. Supporting the ankle,
slide the foot from the shoe.

11. To remove socks, roll the sock down to the ankle, then slip it off the foot.

12. To remove garments that are pulled over the head, first undo buttons, zippers, or other fasteners. Then slip the garment over the patient's stronger arm and shoulder. Raise the patient's head and shoulders, then slip the garment off the patient's weaker arm and shoulder. Pull the garment up over the patient's head.

13. To remove garments that open in front, first undo buttons, zippers, or other fasteners. Then slip the garment off the patient's stronger arm and shoulder. Locking arms with the patient, pull the garment around the patient's back. Slip the garment off the patient's weaker arm and shoulder.

14. To remove garments that open in back, lock arms with the patient and raise the body. Undo buttons, zippers, or other fasteners. Then pull the sides of the garment around to the front of the patient. Lower the patient, and remove the garment.

15. To remove pants or slacks, first undo buttons, zippers, or other fasteners. If the patient can help, ask the patient to lift the hips. Pull the pants down from the hips, and ask the patient to lower the hips. Pull the pants down the legs and over the feet. If the patient cannot help, turn the patient on the weak side, and pull the pants off the stronger side. Then help the patient turn onto the stronger side, and pull the pants off the weak side. Help the patient resume the original position, then pull the pants down the legs and over the feet.

16. Put a clean gown on the patient, or dress the patient in the appropriate clothing.
17. Raise the side rail.
18. Lower the bed to its lowest horizontal position.
19. Adjust the head of the bed to a safe and comfortable position.
20. Make sure the patient can reach the signal light.
21. Open the privacy curtain and the door.
22. Store clothing in the appropriate closet. Put the bath blanket in the laundry bag.
23. Wash your hands.
24. Report to the nurse that you have undressed the patient and any unusual observations.

PROCEDURE: CHANGING THE GOWN OF A PATIENT WITH IV

1. Wash your hands.
2. Check the patient's identification bracelet and speak the patient's name.
3. Explain to the patient that you are going to change the gown.
4. Follow facility policy for asking visitors to leave the room.
5. Obtain a clean gown.
6. Close the privacy curtain.
7. Raise the bed to a high level to ease your body movements.
8. Lower the side rail.
9. Untie the old gown, and loosen it around the patient's body. Cover the patient with the top sheets.
10. Slip the gown off the patient's free arm.

11. Hold the patient's arm that has the IV. Gather the sleeve and slip it over the IV site and tubing. Then place the arm back on the bed, and slip the sleeve off the arm and hand.
12. Keeping the sleeve gathered, slide it along the tubing to the IV bottle.
13. With your other hand, remove the IV bottle from the pole. Slip the bottle and tubing through the sleeve. Be sure the IV bottle remains elevated above the patient's arm at all times.
14. Return the IV bottle to the pole.
15. Reaching under the top linens, remove the old gown.
16. Take the clean gown, and gather the sleeve that will cover the arm with IV.
17. Remove the IV bottle from the pole. Slip the gathered sleeve over the IV bottle, and rehang the bottle on the pole.
18. Slip the sleeve down the tubing and over the patient's hand, IV site, and arm. Adjust the sleeve on the patient's shoulder.
19. Put the other sleeve onto the patient's free arm.
20. Tie the new gown. If the patient prefers, tie the gown only at the neck so that the patient will not be lie on knots.
21. Adjust the gown around the patient's body.
22. Lower the bed to a safe and comfortable position.
23. Raise the side rail.
24. Make sure the patient can reach the signal light.
25. Open the privacy curtain.
26. Place the soiled linen in the laundry bag.

27. Wash your hands.
28. Report to the nurse that you have changed the patient's gown and any unusual observations.

PROCEDURE: GIVING A BACK RUB

1. Wash your hands.
2. Check the patient's identification bracelet and speak the patient's name.
3. Explain to the patient that you are going to give a back rub.
4. Follow facility policy for asking visitors to leave the room.
5. Collect the following equipment and place on the bedside table: bath blanket, towel, lotion, wash basin, bath thermometer.
6. Close the privacy curtain.
7. Raise the bed to a high level to ease your body movements.
8. Lower the rail on the side closest to you.
9. Help the patient turn on the side facing away from you or onto the abdomen.
10. Cover the patient with the bath blanket. Reaching under the bath blanket, pull the top linens down to the patient's hips.
11. Raise the side rail.
12. Fill the basin with 115° F (46° C) water, testing the temperature with the bath thermometer.
13. Place the lotion bottle in the basin, and wash your hands with warm water.
14. Lower the side rail.
15. Pull the bath blanket down to expose the patient's back and buttocks. Untie the gown.

Place a towel lengthwise next to the patient's back.

16. Apply lotion to the lower back.
17. Using firm, long movements, stroke upwards from the buttocks to the neck and shoulders and onto the upper arms. Then stroke back from the arms and shoulders to the buttocks and over both hip areas. Repeat for three minutes or as otherwise directed.
18. For massaging bony areas, use the tips of your index and middle fingers to make circular motions.
19. To knead the skin, pick up tissue between your thumb and fingers. Knead upward from the buttocks to the shoulders, then reverse the direction.
20. Alternate fast, stimulating movements with slow, relaxing ones. Finish the back rub with firm, long strokes.
21. Dry the back with the towel.
22. Tie the gown, and remove the bath blanket.
23. Help the patient return to a comfortable position.
24. Lower the bed to a comfortable and safe position.
25. Raise the side rail.
26. Make sure the patient can reach the signal light.
27. Open the privacy curtain.
28. Clean and return equipment to its proper location, and place soiled linens in the laundry bag.
29. Wash your hands.

30. Report to the nurse that you have given the
    patient a back rub and any unusual
    observations, such as skin irritation or sores.

Principles for Preventing Bedsores

- Change the patient's position a minimum of
  every 2 hours.
- Keep the patient's skin clean and dry at all
  times.
- Give backrubs and skin massages when
  appropriate but not on areas developing sores.
- Avoid vigorous scrubbing or drying of skin
  when bathing.
- Be sure bed linens and the patient's gown are
  clean and dry.
- If ordered, use bed devices such as an
  eggcrate mattress, air mattress, or sheepskin
  pad.
- Report to the nurse any sign of developing
  bedsores.

PROCEDURE: PREVENTING BEDSORES IN THE INCONTINENT PATIENT

1. Wash your hands.
2. Check the patient's identification bracelet and
   speak the patient's name.
3. Explain to the patient that you are going to
   wash the skin.
4. Follow facility policy for asking visitors to leave
   the room.
5. Collect the following equipment and place on
   the bedside table: wash basin, bath
   thermometer, soap and soap dish, toilet
   tissue, lotion, washcloths, disposable gloves,
   towels, bath blanket, bedpan.

6. Close the privacy curtain.
7. Fill the wash basin with 115° F (46° C) water, testing the temperature with the bath thermometer.
8. Raise the bed to a high level to ease your body movements.
9. Lower the rail on the side closest to you.
10. Put on the disposable gloves.
11. Cover the patient with the bath blanket. Reaching under the bath blanket, pull the top sheets down to the patient's feet.
12. Position the patient so that you can reach soiled areas of the skin.
13. Use the toilet tissue to wipe skin that has feces or urine on it. Discard the tissue in the bedpan.
14. Using soap and washcloths, wash the same areas. Rinse with clean water.
15. Using circular motions, dry the areas thoroughly, making sure no moisture remains.
16. Apply lotion to the lower back. Using firm, long movements, stroke upwards from the buttocks to the neck and shoulders. Then reverse the direction of your strokes. Use a washcloth to remove any excess lotion.
17. Change the gown or linens if soiled. Remove the bath blanket
18. Loosen the top sheets around the patient's body to allow air to circulate.
19. Lower the bed to a safe and comfortable level.
20. Raise the side rail.
21. Make sure the patient can reach the signal light.
22. Open the privacy curtain.
23. Empty and clean the bedpan.

24. Clean and return equipment to its proper place, and put soiled linens in the laundry bag. Discard any trash.
25. At least every two hours, change the patient's position and check to see that the patient is still dry. Clean the patient and change the linens as necessary.
26. Wash your hands.
27. Report to the nurse that you have cleaned the patient's skin, the character of the patient's urine or feces, and any signs of skin irritations, sores, or ulcers.

PROCEDURE: CARING FOR BEDSORES

1. Wash your hands.
2. Check the patient's identification bracelet and speak the patient's name.
3. Explain to the patient that you are going to care for the bedsores.
4. Follow facility policy for asking visitors to leave the room.
5. Collect the following equipment: lotion, towels, toilet tissue, bath blanket, disposable gloves.
6. Close the privacy curtain.
7. Raise the bed to a high level to ease your body movements.
8. Lower the rail on the side closest to you.
9. Help the patient move onto the side facing away from you or onto the abdomen.
10. Cover the patient with the bath blanket.
11. Reaching under the bath blanket, pull the top linens down to the patient's knees.
12. Apply lotion to the patient's back. Using firm, long strokes, move from the buttocks to the

neck and shoulders. Use toilet tissue or towel to remove any excess lotion.

13. Gently rub bed sores, starting on the outside of the red area and, using a circular motion, moving to the center.
14. Reaching under the bath blanket, pull the top linens back to their original position.
15. Be sure the bottom linens are tight and free from wrinkles.
16. Check patient's turning schedule, and position the patient on the proper side.
17. Lower the bed to a safe and comfortable position.
18. Raise side rail.
19. Make sure the patient can reach the signal light.
20. Open the privacy curtain.
21. Clean and return equipment to its proper place, and put soiled linens in the laundry bag. Discard any trash.
22. Wash your hands.
23. Report to the nurse that you have cared for the patient's bed sores and any unusual observations.

Chapter 8
Infection Control

This chapter includes information on the following:
   Principles of medical asepsis
   General rules for preventing infection
   Procedure: Handwashing
   General rules for the isolation patient
   Procedure: Putting on a mask
   Procedure: Putting on a gown
   Procedure: Double bagging a gown or linen
   Precautions for the isolation room
   Procedure: Precautions for AIDS patients

Principles of Medical Asepsis

► Medical asepsis is the series of techniques used to prevent all kinds of infection:
   • Infection is the spread of microorganisms from any one person, whether patient or staff or visitors, to another person.
   • Cross-infection is the spread of a microorganism from another patient or staff person to the patient.
   • Reinfection is a second infection of the same patient with the same microorganism.
   • Self-inoculation is the infection of the patient with microorganisms from the patient himself.
   • A nosocomial infection is an infection the patient gets while in the hospital.
   • Secondary infection is one infection on top of another, resulting in a major complication.

▸ There are five main ways to maintain medical asepsis:
  • Cleanliness includes the patient, the unit, all equipment and supplies, your hands and uniform, and anything else that may harbor microorganisms.
  • Disinfection is a method of killing many microorganisms and limiting the growth of others, usually through chemicals, and is used with most supplies and equipment to prevent spread of infection.
  • Sterilization includes methods of killing all microorganisms, such as by steam heat, and is used with all equipment that contacts a wound.
  • Isolation rooms and special techniques are used for patients who have some infections or who are especially susceptible to infection.
  • Gloves, face masks, and gowns are worn when appropriate to prevent the spread of microorganisms.

General Rules for Preventing Infection

■ When washing hands:
  - Wash hands before and after all actions, handling food, and contact with patients.
  - Use the appropriate soap and enough warm running water to lather well; do not use the patient's soap.
  - Because the sink and faucet handles are considered contaminated, start washing over again if your hands contact them; use paper towels to touch the handles.

- Always keep hands lower than the elbows, to prevent unclean water from running back up to clean upper arms.
- When caring for equipment and supplies:
  - Follow accepted facility procedure for disposing of used supplies and dirty linen; do not put dirty linen on the floor.
  - Before reusing equipment, wash it carefully with soap and hot water and then disinfect or sterilize it.
  - Always hold equipment and supplies away from your body and uniform.
  - Carefully pour dirty cleaning water or other fluids into the sink, avoiding splashing.
  - Do not shake out linen or otherwise cause a movement of dust.
- At all times:
  - Wash hands after urination or bowel movement.
  - Wash fresh fruits and vegetables before eating them uncooked.
  - Follow good principles of personal hygiene.
  - Cover nose and mouth when sneezing or coughing; wash hands.
  - Clean from the most clean to least clean area.
  - Do not sit on the patient's bed or otherwise touch your uniform to surfaces that may spread microorganisms.
  - Follow AIDS precautions (see later section) with all patients.

PROCEDURE: HANDWASHING

1. Be sure the appropriate supplies and equipment are at the sink: soap, paper towels, nail file or orange stick, and wastepaper basket.
2. Remove your wristwatch or push it midway to the elbow.
3. Stand so that your uniform does not touch the sink.
4. Use a paper towel to turn on the faucet; adjust to a comfortable warm flow; throw away the paper towel.
5. Keep hands below elbows throughout the process.
6. Wet wrists and hands thoroughly.
7. If using bar soap, rinse the bar thoroughly.
8. Apply soap or detergent and work up a good lather by rubbing palms together.
9. Work the lather over both hands and wrists completely, under nails, and between fingers. Rub tips of fingernails across palms to clean under nails.
10. Rub hands together well, interlace fingers to rub between, and use friction and rotating movements to scrub all skin surfaces to about 2 inches over the wrist thoroughly for 2 minutes.
11. Use orange stick or nail file to clean under nails.
12. Rinse hands and wrists well under running water.
13. Dry hands thoroughly with paper towels.
14. Using a paper towel, turn off the faucet; throw away the paper towel.

General Rules for the Isolation Patient

Note: *There are several kinds of isolation units, such as strict isolation for patients with certain infections to protective isolation for patients susceptible to infection. Always follow specific facility guidelines.*

- Prevent drafts in the room, which may spread microorganisms. Do not shake out linen or otherwise cause dust movement.
- Because the floor is considered contaminated, any object that touches the floor is considered contaminated.
- Use paper towels to handle contaminated objects and to turn faucet handles.
- Double bag and tag all items leaving the room (see procedure for double bagging).
- Wash hands if they touch any contaminated object or surface.
- Avoid touching your own hair, face, or body while giving care in isolation room.
- Inform the nurse if you have any signs of respiratory infection or open skin sores.
- Follow facility policy and correct procedures for wearing gloves, mask, and gown.

PROCEDURE: PUTTING ON A MASK

1. Wash your hands.
2. Take the mask from its container, handling it only by the upper strings; do not touch the part that covers the face.
3. Put the mask over your nose and mouth.

4. Put the top strings over your ears and tie behind your head.
5. Making sure the bottom of the mask is under your chin, tie the lower strings behind your head.
6. If the mask has a metal strip over the nose, mold it into position.
7. Wash your hands.
8. Change the mask if it becomes damp during the time you are providing patient care.
9. To remove the mask, wash hands, untie the bottom ties and then the top ties, and remove the mask while holding the top ties; dispose of the used mask properly.
10. Wash your hands.

PROCEDURE: PUTTING ON A GOWN

1. Roll up your sleeves above the elbow and remove watch and jewelry.
2. Wash your hands.
3. Unfold the clean gown while holding it in front of you; the opening should be at the back.
4. Put your arms through the sleeves.
5. Arrange the gown; be sure it covers your uniform.
6. Tie the strings, or other fastener, at the back of your neck.
7. Pull the gown edges together in back and overlap them such that your uniform is completely covered and the gown fits snugly.
8. Tie the waist strings, or other fastener, at the back.

9. Your hands should still be clean; do not wash them again because the gown sleeves should stay dry.
10. To remove the gown, untie the waist and then the neck strings, pull the gown down from the shoulder by the neck strings, roll it inside out away from you as you remove it, and dispose of it properly.
11. Wash your hands.

PROCEDURE: DOUBLE BAGGING A GOWN OR LINEN

Note: this procedure is used as a precaution for disposing of potentially contaminated linens and gowns from inside an isolation room.

1. Ask another staff person to assist you.
2. Inside the room, place the gown or soiled linen in the linen bag and seal it with tape or string.
3. Ask the other person outside the room to hold open the clean bag with a wide cuff covering the person's hands.
4. Being careful not to touch the outside of the clean bag, put the dirty bag into it.
5. The other staff person now closes and seals the outer bag without touching the inner bag.
6. Put an identifying tag on the other bag and dispose of it according to facility policy.
7. Wash your hands.

Precautions for the Isolation Room

► Follow facility policy for wearing a gown, mask, and gloves.
► Dispose of trash and equipment from the isolation room following facility policy for bagging separate types of materials.
► Take extra care when collecting patient specimens in an isolation room, following facility policy to keep the outside of the container from becoming contaminated or to use double bagging technique.
► After feeding a patient, dispose of leftover food by flushing down the toilet or using a wet garbage bag, and double bag the dishes, utensils, and garbage bags.
► Equipment used for taking vital signs or other procedures performed repeatedly should be left in the isolation room.
► If you must use your watch in the isolation room, put it on a paper towel before entering the room; wash hands before putting it back on, and touch only the top of the paper towel if necessary.

PROCEDURE: PRECAUTIONS FOR AIDS PATIENTS

Note: _The following precautions are recommended for_ _all_ _patients, as you may be providing care for patients with the virus but not known to have AIDS._

1. Take extreme care in handling needles or any other sharp objects that have been in contact with patients.

2. Wear disposable gloves whenever giving care that may involve contact with patients' bodily fluids, including saliva, urine, sneezing, blood, and all other fluids; wear gloves at all times if you have any breaks in your skin.
3. Wash your hands before and after all patient contact and immediately any time they come into contact with patients' bodily fluids.
4. Wear a gown any time your clothing may come into contact patients' bodily fluids.
5. Follow facility policy at all times for cleaning any spilled specimens or blood and for use of disinfectant and sterilization.

Chapter 9
Vital Signs

This chapter includes information on the following:

General Rules for Taking Vital Signs

■ Measure vital signs as ordered, often on a
regular basis.
■ Take care to record vital signs in the
appropriate place with clear handwriting.

Always record a temperature with an O, R, or A beside the number for the site of taking the temperature: Oral, Rectal, or Axillary.

- Report to the nurse any unusual vital signs or any problems you have in measuring them.
- Handle a glass thermometer carefully. If it breaks, clean up the poisonous mercury carefully. Follow facility policy for disinfecting thermometers and their containers. Never use hot water when washing a thermometer.
- Oral temperatures are normally taken. Take a rectal temperature in these situations:
  - Facility policy, for certain patients
  - If the patient's mouth or nose is obstructed by oxygen equipment, nasogastric or other tube, a dressing, or congestion
  - If the patient cannot keep the mouth closed, cannot breathe through the nose, has seizures, is unconscious or disoriented, or is sneezing or coughing
- Do not take a rectal temperature if the patient has a rectal condition, diarrhea, or heart disease.
- Because the axillary temperature is the least accurate, use this site only if the patient cannot tolerate oral or rectal temperature taking. The axilla (armpit) must be dry; do not use this site after bathing the patient.
- Be careful not to confuse an oral thermometer with a rectal thermometer.
- Follow facility policy for use of plastic covers with glass thermometers. Always dispose of the covering properly.

- Be sensitive to the patient's feelings of embarrassment or humiliation when taking a rectal temperature.
- Do not leave the patient alone while a thermometer (of any type) is in place.

PROCEDURE: USING A GLASS THERMOMETER

1. Wash your hands.
2. Obtain a glass thermometer, tissues, and a container of disinfectant solution.
3. Inspect the thermometer for chips, cracks, or other defects. Replace it if necessary.
4. Use your thumb and fingertips to hold the thermometer firmly at the stem. Rinse it in cold water if it was stored in disinfectant solution.
5. To shake the mercury to the lowest point, snap your hand at the wrist while holding the thermometer securely. Repeat until the mercury is below the numbers and lines printed on the thermometer. Be sure to avoid hitting walls, tables, or other furniture.
6. Take the patient's temperature (see following procedure).
7. Shake down the thermometer after use.
8. Wipe the thermometer with tissues and rinse in cold running water.
9. Place the thermometer in the container of disinfectant solution if used.
10. Wash your hands.

PROCEDURE: READING A GLASS THERMOMETER

1.   Wash your hands.
2.   Use your thumb and fingertips to hold the thermometer at the stem.
3.   Holding the thermometer at eye level, slowly turn the thermometer until you can see the mercury.
4.   Look for the scale, a series of lines and numbers.
5.   Look at the end of the mercury, and notice the line at which it ends. On a Centigrade thermometer, each long line measures 1 degree and each small line measures 0.1 degree. On a Fahrenheit thermometer, each long line measures 1 degree and each small line measures 0.2 degrees. Fahrenheit temperatures are always recorded in even tenths of a degree.
6.   Record the temperature on the patient's chart or where otherwise instructed.
7.   Wash your hands.

PROCEDURE: TAKING ORAL TEMPERATURE WITH A GLASS THERMOMETER

1.   Wash your hands.
2.   Check the patient's identification bracelet and speak the patient's name.
3.   Explain that you are going to take the patient's temperature. If the patient has been smoking or drinking hot or cold liquids, wait 10 minutes.
4.   Follow facility policy for asking visitors to leave the room.

5. Obtain an oral thermometer, tissues, container of disinfectant solution, pen.
6. Close the privacy curtain.
7. Inspect the thermometer for chips, cracks, or other defects. Replace it if necessary.
8. Rinse the thermometer under cold running water, and dry it with a tissue.
9. Shake down the mercury. Put plastic disposable sheath, if used, over bulb end.
10. Gently place the thermometer's bulb end under the patient's tongue.
11. Ask the patient to keep the tongue down and lips closed.
12. Leave the thermometer in the patient's mouth for 2-8 minutes, following facility policy.
13. Holding the stem, remove the thermometer from the mouth, remove plastic sheath if used, and gently wipe it with a clean tissue.
14. Read the thermometer.
15. Record the temperature on the patient's chart or where otherwise instructed.
16. Shake down the mercury.
17. Rinse the thermometer under cold running water and place it in a container of disinfectant solution.
18. Make sure the patient is comfortable and can reach the signal light.
19. Open the privacy curtain.
20. Wash your hands.
21. Report to the nurse that you have taken the patient's temperature and any unusual observations.

PROCEDURE: TAKING ORAL TEMPERATURE WITH AN ELECTRONIC THERMOMETER

1. Wash your hands.
2. Check the patient's identification bracelet and speak the patient's name.
3. Explain that you are going to take the patient's temperature. If the patient has been smoking or drinking hot or cold liquids, wait 10 minutes.
4. Follow facility policy for asking visitors to leave the room.
5. Obtain an electronic thermometer, oral probe (usually blue), disposable oral probe covers, pen.
6. Close the privacy curtain.
7. Plug the oral probe into the electronic thermometer, if not already plugged in.
8. Place a disposable probe cover onto the probe.
9. Gently place the probe at the base of the tongue toward the back of the mouth. Hold the probe in place.
10. Ask the patient to keep the tongue down and lips closed.
11. At the sign of a buzzer or flashing or steady light, read the temperature on the digital display.
12. Remove the probe from the patient's mouth.
13. Discard the used probe cover by pressing the eject button.
14. Return the probe to its storage position on the thermometer.
15. Record the temperature on the patient's chart or where otherwise instructed.

16. Make sure the patient is comfortable and can reach the signal light.
17. Open the privacy curtain.
18. Wash your hands.
19. Return the electronic thermometer to its proper location.
20. Report to the nurse that you have taken the patient's temperature and any usual observations.

PROCEDURE: TAKING ORAL TEMPERATURE WITH A DISPOSABLE THERMOMETER

1. Wash your hands.
2. Check the patient's identification bracelet and speak the patient's name.
3. Explain that you are going to take the patient's temperature. If the patient has been smoking or drinking hot or cold liquids, wait 10 minutes.
4. Follow facility policy for asking visitors to leave the room.
5. Obtain a disposable thermometer and a pen.
6. Close the privacy curtain.
7. Unwrap the disposable thermometer.
8. Ask the patient to open the mouth and raise the tongue.
9. Gently position the thermometer at the base of the tongue.
10. Ask the patient to keep the tongue down and lips closed.
11. After 45 seconds, remove the thermometer.
12. To read the temperature, note the location of the last colored dot.
13. Record the temperature on the patient's chart or where otherwise instructed.

14. Dispose of the thermometer.
15. Make sure the patient is comfortable and can reach the signal light.
16. Close the privacy curtain.
17. Wash your hands.
18. Report to the nurse that you have taken the patient's temperature and any unusual observations.

PROCEDURE: TAKING RECTAL TEMPERATURE WITH A GLASS THERMOMETER

1. Wash your hands.
2. Check the patient's identification bracelet and speak the patient's name.
3. Explain to the patient that you are going to take a rectal temperature.
4. Follow facility policy for asking visitors to leave the room.
5. Collect the following equipment: rectal thermometer, tissues, lubricating jelly, disposable gloves, container of disinfectant solution or disposable plastic sheath, pen.
6. Close the privacy curtain.
7. Inspect the thermometer for chips, cracks, or other defects. Replace if necessary.
8. Rinse the thermometer in cold running water, and dry it with tissue.
9. Shake down the mercury. Put on plastic disposable sheath, if used, on bulb end.
10. Lower the backrest and side rail.
11. Help the patient turn onto the side facing away from you. Turn back the top linens to reveal just the buttocks.

12. Put on the disposable gloves.
13. Using a tissue, apply lubricating jelly to the bulb end of the thermometer.
14. Use one hand to raise the upper buttock and expose the anus. With other hand, gently insert the bulb of the thermometer 1 inch through the patient's anus and into the rectum. Do not use force.
15. Hold the thermometer in place for 2-3 minutes, following facility policy. Never leave a patient with a thermometer in the rectum.
16. Remove the thermometer from the rectum.
17. Remove plastic sheath, if used. Wipe the thermometer with tissues.
18. Wipe the anal area with tissues to remove excess lubricating jelly. Pull up the top linens to cover the patient.
19. Raise the side rail.
20. Read the temperature.
21. Record the temperature, with an "R" to indicate it was taken rectally, on the patient's chart or where otherwise instructed.
22. Shake down the mercury.
23. Rinse and wash the thermometer. Place it in a container of disinfectant solution.
24. Raise the backrest to a comfortable and safe position.
25. Make sure the patient can reach the signal light.
26. Open the privacy curtain.
27. Return equipment to its proper location, and discard any trash.
28. Wash your hands.

29. Report to the nurse that you have taken the patient's rectal temperature and any unusual observations.

PROCEDURE: TAKING RECTAL TEMPERATURE WITH AN ELECTRONIC THERMOMETER

1. Wash your hands.
2. Check the patient's identification bracelet and speak the patient's name.
3. Explain to the patient that you are going to take a rectal temperature.
4. Follow facility policy for asking visitors to leave the room.
5. Collect the following equipment: electronic thermometer, rectal probe (usually red), disposable probe covers, tissues, lubricating jelly, disposable gloves, pen.
6. Close the privacy curtain.
7. Plug the rectal probe into the electronic thermometer, if it is not already plugged in.
8. Place a disposable probe cover onto the probe.
9. Lower the backrest and side rail.
10. Help the patient turn onto the side facing away from you. Turn back the top linens to reveal just the buttocks.
11. Put on the disposable gloves.
12. Using a tissue, apply lubricating jelly to the end of the probe cover.

13. Use one hand to raise the upper buttock and expose the anus. With the other hand, gently insert the probe through the patient's anus and 1/2 inch into the rectum. Hold the probe in place.
14. At the sign of a buzzer or flashing or steady light, read the temperature on the digital display.
15. Remove the probe from the patient's rectum.
16. Discard the used probe by pressing the eject button.
17. Return the probe to the storage position on the thermometer.
18. Wipe the anal area with tissues to remove excess lubricating jelly. Pull up the top linens to cover the patient.
19. Raise the side rail.
20. Record the temperature, with an "R" to indicate it was taken rectally, on the patient's chart or where otherwise instructed.
21. Raise the backrest to a comfortable and safe position.
22. Make sure the patient can reach the signal light.
23. Open the privacy curtain.
24. Return equipment to its proper location, and discard any trash.
25. Wash your hands.
26. Report to the nurse that you have taken the patient's rectal temperature, and any unusual observations.

PROCEDURE: TAKING AXILLARY TEMPERATURE WITH A GLASS THERMOMETER

1. Wash your hands.
2. Check the patient's identification bracelet and speak the patient's name.
3. Explain to the patient that you are going to take an axillary, or underarm, temperature.
4. Follow facility policy for asking visitors to leave the room.
5. Obtain an oral thermometer, tissue, container of disinfectant solution or disposable plastic sheath, towel, pen.
6. Close the privacy curtain.
7. Inspect the thermometer for chips, cracks, or other defects. Replace it if necessary.
8. Rinse the thermometer under cold running water, and dry it with a tissue.
9. Shake down the thermometer. Put the disposable plastic sheath, if used, over the bulb end.
10. Remove one of the patient's arms from the sleeve of the gown.
11. Dry the axilla, or armpit, with the towel.
12. Position the bulb of the thermometer in the center of the armpit.
13. To hold the thermometer in place, position the patient's arm over the chest. If the patient cannot help, hold the thermometer and arm in place yourself.
14. Leave the thermometer in place for 10 minutes. Stay with the patient while waiting.

15. Holding the stem, remove the thermometer from the armpit, remove disposable plastic sheath if used, and wipe it with a tissue.
16. Read the thermometer.
17. Record the temperature, with an "A" to indicate it is axillary, on the patient's chart or where otherwise instructed.
18. Put the sleeve of the gown back on the patient's arm.
19. Raise the backrest to a comfortable and safe position.
20. Make sure the patient can reach the signal light.
21. Shake down the mercury.
22. Rinse the thermometer under cold running water and place it in a container of disinfectant solution.
23. Open the privacy curtain.
24. Return equipment to its proper location, place the soiled towel in the laundry bag, and discard any trash.
25. Wash your hands.
26. Report to the nurse that you have taken the patient's axillary temperature and any unusual observations.

PROCEDURE: TAKING AXILLARY TEMPERATURE WITH AN ELECTRONIC THERMOMETER

1. Wash your hands.
2. Check the patient's identification bracelet and speak the patient's name.
3. Explain to the patient that you are going to take an axillary, or underarm, temperature.

4. Follow facility policy for asking visitors to leave the room.
5. Obtain an electronic thermometer, oral probe (usually blue), disposable probe covers, towel, pen.
6. Close the privacy curtain.
7. Plug the oral probe into the electronic thermometer, if it not already plugged in.
8. Place a disposable probe cover onto the probe.
9. Remove one of the patient's arms from the sleeve of the gown.
10. Dry the axilla, or armpit, with the towel.
11. Place the covered probe in the center of the patient's armpit.
12. Place the patient's arm over the chest. Hold the probe in place.
13. At the sign of a buzzer or flashing or steady light, remove the probe and read the temperature on the digital display.
14. Record the temperature, with an "A" to indicate it is axillary, on the patient's chart or where otherwise instructed.
15. Discard the used probe by pressing the eject button.
16. Return the probe to the storage area on the thermometer.
17. Put the sleeve of the gown back on the patient's arm.
18. Adjust the headrest to a comfortable and safe position.
19. Make sure the patient can reach the signal light.
20. Open the privacy curtain.

21. Return equipment to its proper location, place the towel in the laundry bag, and discard any trash.
22. Wash your hands.
23. Report to the nurse that you have taken the patient's axillary temperature and any unusual observations.

PROCEDURE: MEASURING THE RADIAL PULSE

1. Wash your hands.
2. Check the patient's identification bracelet and speak the patient's name.
3. Explain that you are going to take the patient's pulse.
4. Follow facility policy for asking visitors to leave the room.
5. Obtain a watch with a second hand and a pen.
6. Close the privacy curtain.
7. Ask the patient to sit or lie down. Make sure the patient's arm is well-supported and at ease.
8. To find the pulse, place your middle three fingers on the patient's inner wrist below the thumb. Press lightly. Do not use your own thumb, for it has its own pulse.
9. Note the pulse's rhythm, whether it is steady or irregular and whether it is strong or weak.
10. If the pulse is strong and steady, count the pulse for 30 seconds, using your watch. Multiply the number of beats by two. If the pulse is weak or irregular, count the beats for a full minute.

11. Record the pulse on the patient's chart or where otherwise indicated. Also note the pulse's strength and regularity.
12. Adjust the headrest to a comfortable and safe position.
13. Make sure the patient can reach the signal light.
14. Open the privacy curtain.
15. Wash your hands.
16. Report to the nurse that you have taken the patient's pulse. Be sure to note and report a pulse rate under 60 or over 100, the pulse's strength, and its regularity.

PROCEDURE: MEASURING THE APICAL PULSE

1. Wash your hands.
2. Check the patient's identification bracelet and speak the patient's name.
3. Explain that you are going to check the patient's apical pulse.
4. Follow facility policy for asking visitors to leave.
5. Obtain a stethoscope, a watch with second hand, antiseptic swabs, pen.
6. Close the privacy curtain.
7. Wipe the earpieces and diaphragm (or bell) of the stethoscope with the antiseptic swabs.
8. Help the patient sit or lie down.
9. Uncover the nipple area of the left chest, taking care not to overexpose the patient.
10. Warm the diaphragm of the stethoscope by holding it in your hand.
11. Place the earpieces in your ears.

12. To locate the apical pulse, place the diaphragm about 1 inch below and just to the right of the patient's left nipple.
13. Count the pulse for one full minute, noting its regularity. Each "lub-dub" sound counts as one pulse.
14. Remove the stethoscope and cover the patient.
15. Record the apical pulse, with an "Ap" to indicate it was taken apically, on the patient's chart or where otherwise instructed.
16. Adjust the backrest to a comfortable and safe position.
17. Make sure the patient can reach the signal light.
18. Open the privacy curtain.
19. Wipe the earpieces and diaphragm of the stethoscope with antiseptic swabs.
20. Return equipment to its proper location, and discard any trash.
21. Report to the nurse that you have taken the patient's apical pulse. Be sure to note and report a pulse under 60 or above 100, the pulse's strength, and its regularity.

PROCEDURE: MEASURING A PULSE DEFICIT

1. Ask a nurse or nursing assistant to help you.
2. Wash your hands.
3. Check the patient's identification bracelet and speak the patient's name.
4. Explain that you are going to check the patient's radial and apical pulse.
5. Follow facility policy for asking visitors to leave the room.

6. Obtain a stethoscope, antiseptic swabs, a watch with second hand, pen.
7. Close the privacy curtain.
8. Wipe the earpieces and diaphragm (or bell) or the stethoscope with the antiseptic swabs.
9. Help the patient sit or lie down.
10. Uncover the nipple area of the left chest, taking care not to overexpose the patient.
11. Warm the diaphragm by holding it in your hand.
12. Place the earpieces in your ears.
13. Locate the apical pulse. At the same time, your partner should locate the radial pulse.
14. Signal your partner to start counting the pulse.
15. Count the pulse for one full minute.
16. Signal your partner to stop counting.
17. Remove the stethoscope and cover the patient.
18. Record the radial and apical pulses on the patient's chart or where otherwise instructed. To find the pulse deficit, subtract the radial pulse from the apical pulse. Note the pulse's strength and regularity.
19. Adjust the backrest to a comfortable and safe position.
20. Make sure the patient can reach the signal light.
21. Open the privacy curtain.
22. Wipe the earpieces and diaphragm of the stethoscope with antiseptic swabs.
23. Return equipment to its proper place, and discard any trash.
24. Report to the nurse that you have measured the patient's pulse deficit. Be sure to note the apical and radial pulse rates, the pulse deficit,

and pulse's strength and regularity, and any unusual observations.

PROCEDURE: MEASURING RESPIRATIONS

1. Wash your hands.
2. Obtain a watch with second hand and a pen.
3. Check the patient's identification bracelet and speak the patient's name.
4. Follow facility policy for asking visitors to leave the room.
5. Respiration is measured at the same time as pulse. Do not tell the patient that you are measuring respiration. If you have taken a radial pulse, keep your hand on the patient's wrist. If you have taken an apical pulse, keep the stethoscope on the patient's chest.
6. Note whether the patient's breathing is painful or difficult, and note the depth and regularity of the respirations.
7. Start counting when the patient's chest rises. One rise and one fall of the chest counts as one respiration.
8. If the respirations are regular, count for 30 seconds, using your watch.   Multiply the number of respirations by two. If the respirations are irregular, count for a full minute.
9. Record the respiration rate on the patient's chart or where otherwise instructed.
10. Adjust the backrest to a comfortable and safe position.
11. Make sure the patient can reach the signal light.
12. Wash your hands.

13. Report to the nurse that you have measured the patient's respirations. Note the respiration rate, and the depth, regularity, and ease of respiration, and any unusual observations.

PROCEDURE: TAKING A BLOOD PRESSURE

1. Wash your hands.
2. Check the patient's identification bracelet and speak the patient's name.
3. Explain that you are going to take the patient's blood pressure.
4. Follow facility policy for asking visitors to leave the room.
5. Obtain a stethoscope, sphygmomanometer (blood pressure cuff), antiseptic swabs, pen.
6. Close the privacy curtain.
7. Help the patient sit or lie down.
8. Wipe the earpieces of the stethoscope with an antiseptic swab. Place the earpieces in your ears.
9. Push the patient's sleeve above the elbow. Position the arm so that it is level with the heart and the palm is facing upward.
10. Stand no more than 3 feet away from the sphygmomanometer. A mercury model should be at eye level, while the aneroid model should be in front of you.
11. Squeeze any remaining air out of the cuff. Close the bulb valve.
12. Wrap the cuff around the patient's arm at least 1 inch above the elbow. The cuff should be snug but not tight.

13. With your fingertips, find the patient's brachial artery at the inside of the elbow. The diaphragm of the stethoscope will be positioned here.
14. Locate the radial artery. Inflate the cuff until you cannot feel the radial pulse. Then inflate the cuff 30 mm Hg more.
15. Place the diaphragm of the stethoscope over the brachial artery.
16. Deflate the cuff evenly by turning the valve counterclockwise. Deflate it at a rate of 2 to 4 mm per second.
17. As you deflate the cuff, watch the scale. The first sound you hear will indicate the systolic pressure.
18. Continue deflating the cuff. When the sound disappears, note the diastolic pressure.
19. Deflate the cuff completely. Remove it from the patient's arm.
20. Record the blood pressure on the patient's chart or where otherwise instructed.
21. Wipe the earpieces and diaphragm of the stethoscope with the antiseptic swabs.
22. Adjust the backrest to a safe and comfortable position.
23. Make sure the patient can reach the signal light.
24. Open the privacy curtain.
25. Return equipment to its proper location, and discard any trash.
26. Wash your hands.
27. Report to the nurse that you have taken the patient's blood pressure and any unusual observations.

Chapter 10
Nutrition, Diet, and Fluids

This chapter includes information on the following:
  Principles of special diets
  General rules for feeding patients
  Procedure: Preparing the patient for meals
  Procedure: Serving a meal
  Procedure: Feeding the patient
  Procedure: Feeding by mouth using bulb syringe
  Procedure: Providing fresh water
  Principles of fluid balance
  Procedure: Measuring fluid intake and output
  General rules for nasogastric tube care

Principles of Special Diets

▶ The facility's regular diet for patients is nutritionally complete, but the doctor may prescribe a special diet for a patient for a variety of conditions.

▶ The special diet may be restricted in one or more of the following ways:
  • Low-sodium (salt) or sodium-free diet
  • Low- (or high-) calorie diet
  • Low-residue (bulk) or high-fiber diet
  • Clear liquid diet
  • Soft foods only
  • Bland (low in spices) diet
  • Diabetic diet

- Low-fat, low-cholesterol diet
- High-protein diet
- High-iron diet

▸ The doctor may order restricted fluids (specifying the maximum daily quantity allowed) or forced fluids (increased consumption of fluids).

▸ The doctor may order the patient to be temporarily NPO (nothing per oral--nothing by mouth), not allowed either to drink or eat.

▸ Your role in all special dietary situations is to follow the orders exactly, without allowing exceptions, and to be empathetic and supportive for the patient who may not easily accept the restrictions. Help the patient realize that any dietary change will have positive effect on the patient's health.

General Rules for Feeding Patients

■ Try to make the environment for eating attractive, pleasant, and appealing; remove any negative distractions such as a bedpan.

■ If the patient is not on a restricted diet, try to arrange to have any requested foods served to the patient.

■ Serve food trays promptly while food is at the best temperature.

■ Because patients who are unable to feed themselves may be depressed or angry, be friendly, encouraging, and patient.

■ Never rush any patient through a meal, particularly one whom you are feeding.

- Be sensitive to a patient's handicap; with a blind patient, describe the placement of food on the tray or plate, by comparing position to the face of a clock.
- Prepare the patient (see following procedure) before you bring the food tray.
- Be sure to follow facility policy and any dietary restrictions when giving snacks between meals.
- Unless the patient's fluid intake is restricted, be sure the water pitcher is always full and provide ice if allowed.
- If a patient is fed through a nasogastric tube (gavage feeding) or through an IV, be sure to follow orders carefully and exactly when assisting.
- Serve only one tray at a time to prevent contamination from one tray to another.

PROCEDURE: PREPARING THE PATIENT FOR MEALS

1. Check the patient's identification bracelet and speak the patient's name.
2. Explain that you are going to prepare the patient for a meal.
3. Wash your hands.
4. Follow facility policy for asking visitors to leave the room.
5. Collect the following equipment: bedpan or urinal, basin with warm wash water, washcloth, soap, towel, toothbrush and toothpaste, and the patient's robe and slippers.
6. Close the privacy curtain and/or room door.

7. Assist the patient as needed with brushing teeth.
8. Offer the urinal or bedpan or help the patient to the bathroom; help the patient put on robe and slippers.
9. Ask or help the patient to wash hands.
10. Adjust the bed, if allowed, so that the patient can sit up comfortably, or let the patient sit in the chair beside the bed.
11. Clean and adjust the overbed table for the patient. Be sure the signal light is within reach.
12. Be sure the patient is comfortable. Straighten up the area if necessary. Return equipment to its place.
13. Open the privacy curtain.
14. Wash your hands.
15. Report to the nurse that the patient is ready for the meal.

PROCEDURE: SERVING A MEAL

1. Wash your hands.
2. Check the patient's identification bracelet and speak the patient's name. Assist the patient to a comfortable eating position.
3. Explain that you are going to serve the patient the meal.
4. Check the tray and menu card to make sure it is the correct food for the patient. Carry the tray at waist height, not shoulder height near the hair.
5. If the patient cannot eat at this time, take the tray away to keep it warm.

6. Put the tray on the overbed table and adjust its height to a comfortable level.
7. Arrange the silverware and dishes for the patient and provide drinking water. Assist with opening milk cartons, pouring a drink, cutting meat, opening food covers, and so on.
8. Give any help that the patient may need with the food.
9. If the patient will eat unassisted, leave the room.
10. Return and remove the tray.
11. If ordered, record what the patient has eaten and drunk.
12. Assist the patient with oral hygiene (see Chapter 7).
13. Tidy the room and clean any spilled food.
14. Help the patient to a position of comfort and move the signal light within reach.
15. Raise the bed side rails if appropriate. Wash your hands.
16. Report to the nurse that you have served the meal, the patient's appetite level, and any observations.

PROCEDURE: FEEDING THE PATIENT

1. Wash your hands.
2. Check the patient's identification bracelet and speak the patient's name. Assist the patient to a comfortable eating position.
3. Explain that you are going to feed the patient the meal.

4. Check the tray and menu card to make sure it is the correct food for the patient. Carry the tray at waist height, not shoulder height near the hair.
5. If the patient cannot eat at this time, take the tray away to keep it warm.
6. Put the tray on the overbed table where the patient can see it and at a comfortable working height.
7. Position a napkin under the patient's chin and across the chest.
8. If the patient is visually impaired, describe the food.
9. Prepare the food and liquid. Add salt or pepper if allowed and if the patient requests it.
10. Use a straw for liquids if the patient cannot drink from a cup. Use a separate straw for each liquid. Warn the patient about hot foods or liquids.
11. For safety reasons, always use only a spoon to feed the patient. Fill the spoon only part way. Give the food from the spoon's tip.
12. Feed foods in the order requested by the patient, or alternate foods in the order one would normally eat. Alternate between solids and liquids. Encourage the patient to chew food thoroughly, and do not rush the patient. You may converse pleasantly with the patient.
13. Wipe the patient's mouth as necessary.
14. Encourage the patient to finish the meal, but stop feeding when the patient requests it.
15. When finished, help the patient wipe the mouth with the napkin.
16. Remove the tray.

17. If ordered, record what the patient has eaten and drunk.
18. Assist the patient with oral hygiene (see Chapter 7).
19. Tidy the room and clean any spilled food.
20. Help the patient to a position of comfort and move the signal light within reach.
21. Raise the bed side rails if appropriate. Wash your hands.
22. Report to the nurse that you have served the meal, the patient's appetite level, and any observations.

PROCEDURE: FEEDING BY MOUTH USING BULB SYRINGE

1. With premixed foods kept cold, remove the food at least 30 minutes in advance or warm it when ready to feed the patient.
2. Wash your hands.
3. Check the patient's identification bracelet and speak the patient's name. Assist the patient to a comfortable eating position.
4. Explain that you are going to feed the patient. Explain why the bulb syringe is being used.
5. Check the tray and equipment to make sure it is the correct food for the patient.
6. Put the tray on the overbed table at a comfortable working height.
7. Position a napkin under the patient's chin and across the chest.
8. Fill the bulb syringe by squeezing the bulb and then releasing pressure on it with the tube opening in the food.

9. Tell the patient you will start the feeding now, a little at a time, giving plenty of time to swallow.
10. Put the syringe tip into the patient's mouth at one side. Squeeze very slowly and give no more than 15 cc between swallows. Give the patient time to swallow.
11. If any of the liquid food spills over the patient's lips, wipe the patient's mouth.
12. Encourage the patient to take the complete amount of food, and do not rush the patient. You may converse pleasantly with the patient.
13. Encourage the patient to finish the meal, but stop feeding when the patient requests it.
14. When finished, wipe the patient's mouth with the napkin.
15. Remove the equipment and tray.
16. If ordered, record how much of the food mixture the patient has taken.
17. Assist the patient with oral hygiene (see Chapter 7).
18. Tidy the room.
19. Help the patient to a position of comfort and move the signal light within reach.
20. Raise the bed side rails if appropriate. Wash your hands.
21. Report to the nurse that you have fed the patient, the patient's appetite level, and any observations.

PROCEDURE: PROVIDING FRESH WATER

1. Follow the procedure used in your facility.
2. Wash your hands.

3. Gather the appropriate equipment, such as cart, ice chest with cubes and cover, ice scoop, disposable cups, water pitcher filled with water, straws, and paper towels.
4. Move the cart outside the patient's room.
5. Check the orders for the patient. Some patients may be NPO (nothing by mouth), on restricted amounts of water, or not allowed ice.
6. Check the patient's identification bracelet and speak the patient's name.
7. Empty the patient's previous water pitcher into the bathroom sink.
8. Refill the pitcher halfway from the tap at the sink or the pitcher on the cart.
9. Using the scoop, fill the water pitcher rest of the way with ice cubes.
10. Put the pitcher on the overbed table within the patient's reach.
11. Put one or more disposable cups and straws beside the pitcher.
12. Dispose of used cups and wipe up any spills with paper towels.
13. Offer to pour the patient a cup of water.
14. Wash your hands.
15. Move the cart to the next patient's room and repeat the procedure.
16. Report to the nurse that you have provided fresh water and any observations.

Principles of Fluid Balance

▸ Because water is needed for body functions and is normally lost through elimination, perspiration, and respiration, fluid intake must balance the amount used or lost.

- In many illnesses the doctor may order restricted fluids or forced fluids.
- If the doctor or nurse orders the patient's fluid intake and output to be measured, this information is needed for the patient's medical treatment.
- Measurements of intake and output must be accurate.
- Fluid intake includes IV liquids, tube feedings, and soft foods such as ice cream and pudding.
- Fluid output includes urine, vomit, diarrhea, and colostomy and wound drainage.
- Intake and output records are kept at the patient's bedside. Each amount is measured and recorded at the time of intake or output.
- Explain the purpose of intake and output records to the patient's to assure the patient's understanding and cooperation. Some patients may be allowed to measure and record intake.
- Teach patients to use the bedpan or urinal and not to use the toilet; patients should not put tissues in the urinal or bedpan.

PROCEDURE: MEASURING FLUID INTAKE AND OUTPUT

1. Explain to the patient why and how you will be measuring the intake and output of fluids.
2. Gather the following equipment at the bedside: the intake and output record sheet, pen, and graduate (measuring cup marked in cc's).
3. Have the patient take fluids only from containers of known size.

4. Measure and record intake after every meal and, for water, periodically throughout the shift following facility policy:
    a. Pour the fluid remaining in a container into the graduate to measure the leftover amount.
    b. Place the graduate on a flat surface and read the measurement at eye level.
    c. Subtract this amount from the amount of fluid originally in the container. (If the amount that fits in the container is unknown, fill it with water and measure it with the graduate. Record this information on the intake out output record sheet for future reference.)
    d. Determine the amounts taken in from other containers as well, and add them for the total amount.
    e. Record the total fluid intake in cc and the time on the intake and output record.
5. Measure the patient's urinary output (and vomiting or diarrhea or colostomy drainage by similar method) after every voiding:
    a. Wash your hands.
    b. Carefully pour the urine from the urinal or bedpan into the graduate.
    c. Place the graduate on a flat surface and read the measurement at eye level.
    d. Record the amount and the time on the intake and output record sheet.
    e. Wash and rinse the graduate and urinal or bedpan and put them in appropriate places.
6. Wash your hands.
7. Report to the nurse that you have measured the intake or output and any observations.

General Rules for Nasogastric Tube Care

- The doctor may order a patient to be fed by nasogastric tube, also called gavage feeding, because of a medical condition. Always follow orders exactly when caring for a patient with a nasogastric tube in place.
- Be careful never to pull on the tube when helping a patient move.
- Reduce the pressure on the tube by keeping it fastened to the patient's gown.
- Handle the tube carefully when helping the patient bathe. Keep the tube clean and the patient's nostril area free of mucus.
- Report to the nurse immediately any gagging or vomiting by the patient.
- Follow the nurse's orders and facility policy to assist with nasogastric tube feeding, such as watching the patient to ensure the formula drains slowly and evenly into the patient's stomach. Report to the nurse if the tube seems blocked.
- Use formula that has warmed to room temperature.
- Typically a glass of water is poured into the feeding container and allowed to drain slowly through the nasogastric tube after the feeding. Report to the nurse how much water and formula was fed, how the patient responded, and any observations.

Chapter 11
Elimination

This chapter includes information on the following:
General rules for urinary elimination
Procedure: Helping the patient use a bedside commode
Procedure: Helping the patient with a bedpan
Procedure: Helping the patient with a urinal
General rules for catheter care
Procedure: Caring for the patient on a catheter
Procedure: Emptying a urinary drainage bag
General rules for collecting urine specimens
Procedure: Collecting a routine urine specimen
Procedure: Collecting a urine specimen from a child or infant
Procedure: Collecting a clean-catch urine specimen
Procedure: Collecting a 24-hour urine specimen
Procedure: Collecting a double-voided urine specimen
Procedure: Performing the Testape urine test
Procedure: Performing the Clinitest urine test
Procedure: Performing the Acetest urine test
Procedure: Performing the Ketostix urine test
Procedure: Performing urine straining
General rules for bowel elimination
General rules for giving an enema
Procedure: Giving a cleansing enema
Procedure: Giving a commercial enema
Procedure: Giving an oil retention enema
Procedure: Rectal tube use
Procedure: Inserting a rectal suppository
Procedure: Collecting a stool specimen

General rules for ostomy care
Procedure: Ostomy care

General Rules for Urinary Elimination

- For patients who cannot leave the bed easily to reach the bathroom, a urinal (for the male patient) or bedpan (for female patient) is used for urination.
- Offer the patient the urinal or bedpan periodically when providing care, and bring it as soon as requested.
- Be sure the urinal or bedpan is warm before offering it.
- Give the patient privacy, or stay nearby if the patient may need assistance.
- Always give the patient sufficient time for urination; never rush the patient.
- After urination, cover the urinal or bedpan and remove it to the bathroom immediately after use; measure urine if the patient is on a intake and output record (see Chapter 10).
- Assist the patient with perineal care if needed (see Chapter 7).
- After urination, always give the patient a washcloth to wash the hands.
- It is generally recommended that you wear disposable gloves when performing procedures involving the patient's urine.

PROCEDURE: HELPING THE PATIENT USE A BEDSIDE COMMODE

1. Explain to the patient what you are going to do.
2. Check the patient's identification bracelet and speak the patient's name.
3. Follow facility policy for asking visitors to leave the room.
4. Close the privacy curtain.
5. Collect the following equipment: portable bedside commode, toilet tissue, bath blanket, basin of warm water, soap, towel, and disposable gloves.
6. Wash your hands.
7. Position the commode beside the bed and open the cover; put a bedpan under the seat or open the container provided with the commode.
8. Lower the bed side rail, and help the patient to the side of the bed to put on slippers and (optionally) robe.
9. Help the patient to the commode. Provide the bath blanket to cover the patient's lap.
10. Make sure the patient can reach the toilet tissue and signal light.
11. Tell the patient to signal for assistance or when finished.
12. Wash your hands.
13. Leave the room and close the door.
14. After the patient signals, return to the room.
15. Wash your hands and put on disposable gloves.

16. If the patient needs help in cleaning the genital (or rectal) area, assist as needed (see Chapter 7 procedures).
17. Help the patient back to bed and remove robe and slippers.
18. Using the basin of water and soap, help the patient wash the hands.
19. Close the commode cover; cover and take the container or bedpan to the bathroom.
20. Check the urine and/or feces for unusual appearance.
21. Measure the urine output if appropriate (see Chapter 10 procedure) or collect specimen if ordered (see later procedure).
22. Empty the urine and/or feces into the toilet.
23. Follow facility policy for cleaning and disinfecting the bedpan or container; return it to its proper place.
24. Clean the commode and return it to its proper place.
25. Make sure the patient is comfortable and the signal light is within reach.
26. Raise the side rail if appropriate.
27. Open the privacy curtain.
28. Dispose of dirty linen or towels.
29. Remove and dispose of your gloves.
30. Wash your hands.
31. Report to the nurse that the patient has urinated and/or defecated and any unusual observations.

PROCEDURE: HELPING THE PATIENT WITH A BEDPAN

1. Ask if the patient would like the bedpan.
2. Check the patient's identification bracelet and speak the patient's name.
3. Follow facility policy for asking visitors to leave the room.
4. Close the privacy curtain.
5. Collect the following equipment: bedpan and cover, toilet tissue, basin of warm water, soap, towel, paper towels, and disposable gloves.
6. Wash your hands.
7. Raise the bed to a high level to ease your body movements.
8. Warm the bedpan by running warm water over it; dry it with paper towels.
9. Position the patient on the back, if not already.
10. Fold back the bed linen out of the way but keep the lower body covered. Lower the bed side rail.
11. Show the patient how to bend the knees and raise the hips; if needed, assist by sliding one hand under the patient's lower back to help lift the buttocks. Slide the bedpan under the patient.
12. If the patient cannot lift the buttocks for the bedpan, turn the patient on the side facing away from you, position the bedpan against the buttocks, and turn the patient back onto the back with bedpan in place.
13. Fold the bed linens back over the patient.
14. Raise the head of the bed or backrest so that the patient is in a sitting position.

15. Make sure the patient can reach the toilet tissue and signal light.
16. Raise the side rail.
17. Tell the patient to signal for assistance or when finished.
18. Wash your hands.
19. Leave the room and close the door.
20. After the patient signals, return to the room.
21. Wash your hands and put on disposable gloves.
22. Lower the side rail.
23. Help the patient raise hips and remove the bedpan. If the patient cannot help, hold the bedpan in place and turn the patient onto the side away from you off the bedpan.
24. Cover the bedpan.
25. If the patient needs help in cleaning the genital or rectal area, assist as needed (see Chapter 7 procedures).
26. Using the basin of water and soap, help the patient wash the hands.
27. Take the bedpan to the bathroom.
28. Check the urine and/or feces for unusual appearance.
29. Measure the urine output if appropriate (see Chapter 10 procedure) or collect specimen if ordered (see later procedure).
30. Empty the urine and/or feces into the toilet.
31. Follow facility policy for cleaning and disinfecting the bedpan; return it to its proper place.
32. Lower the bed to its lowest horizontal position. Lower the head of the bed or the backrest for the patient's comfort and raise the side rail if appropriate.

33. Make sure the patient is comfortable and the signal light is within reach.
34. Open the privacy curtain.
35. Dispose of dirty linen or towels.
36. Remove and dispose of your gloves. Wash your hands.
37. Report to the nurse that the patient has urinated and/or defecated and any unusual observations.

PROCEDURE: HELPING THE PATIENT WITH A URINAL

1. Ask if the male patient would like the urinal.
2. Check the patient's identification bracelet and speak his name.
3. Follow facility policy for asking visitors to leave the room.
4. Close the privacy curtain.
5. Collect the following equipment: urinal and cover, toilet tissue, basin of warm water, soap, towel, paper towels, waterproof pad, and disposable gloves.
6. Raise the head of the bed or backrest so that the patient is in a sitting position.
7. Give the patient the urinal and remind him to tilt it to avoid spilling urine. Put a waterproof pad under the urinal. If necessary for a helpless patient, put on the disposable gloves and position the urinal between the patient's legs and position the patient's penis into it.
8. Make sure the patient can reach the signal light.
9. Tell the patient to signal for assistance or when finished.

10. Wash your hands.
11. Leave the room and close the door.
12. After the patient signals, return to the room.
13. Wash your hands and put on disposable gloves.
14. Take the urinal from the patient, cover it, and take it to the bathroom.
15. If the patient needs help in cleaning the genital area, assist as needed (see Chapter 7 procedures).
16. Using the basin of water and soap, help the patient wash the hands.
17. Check the urine for unusual appearance.
18. Measure the urine output if appropriate (see Chapter 10 procedure) or collect specimen if ordered (see later procedure).
19. Empty the urine into the toilet.
20. Follow facility policy for cleaning and disinfecting the urinal; return it to its proper place.
21. Lower the head of the bed or backrest for the patient's comfort. Make sure the signal light is within reach.
22. Open the privacy curtain.
23. Dispose of dirty linen or towels.
24. Remove and dispose of your gloves. Wash your hands.
25. Report to the nurse that the patient has urinated and any unusual observations.

General Rules for Catheter Care

- Frequently observe the catheter system to be sure urine can flow freely through it. Prevent kinks in the tubing, and at all times make sure the collection bag is below the patient's body level.
- Keep the catheter taped to the patient's thigh to stabilize it and prevent tugging from tube movement.
- Follow facility policy to provide care for the catheter once or twice daily (see following procedure).
- Empty the collection bag at the ordered times and measure the urine collected. Observe the urine's color and clarity and report to the nurse anything unusual.
- Report to the nurse any patient problems such as pain or burning feelings.

PROCEDURE: CARING FOR THE PATIENT ON A CATHETER

1. Wash your hands.
2. Check the patient's identification bracelet and speak the patient's name.
3. Explain to the patient what you are going to do.
4. Follow facility policy for asking visitors to leave the room. Close the privacy curtain.
5. Collect the following equipment: catheter care kit, disposable bed protector, equipment and supplies for perineal care (Chapter 7), bath blanket, and disposable gloves.

6. Raise the bed to a high level to ease your body movements. Lower the side rail.
7. Cover the patient with a bath blanket and fold the bed linens down to the foot of the bed.
8. Follow the procedure to give the patient perineal care (Chapter 7)
9. Helping the patient raise the buttocks as you would with a bedpan, put the bed protector under the patient's buttocks.
10. Open the catheter care kit. Put on disposable gloves.
11. Fold back one corner of the bath blanket to expose the genital area.
12. Take the applicators from the catheter care kit; be sure they are covered with antiseptic.
   For the male:
   a. Retract the foreskin of an uncircumcised male.
   b. Look for any irritated areas or unusual appearance of the penis.
   c. Apply antiseptic solution to the head of the penis; discard the applicator.
   For the female:
   a. Carefully separate the labia with thumb and index finger.
   b. Look for any irritated areas or unusual appearance of the genital area.
   c. Apply antiseptic solution to the labia and area where the catheter tube enters the urethra; discard the applicator.
13. Apply antiseptic solution to about 4 inches of the catheter tube near the insertion; discard the applicator.

14. Check that the tubing is taped securely to the patient's thigh, coiled loosely, and not kinked between the catheter and collection bag.
15. Remove the bed protector. Remove the bath blanket. Fold the bed linen back into place over the patient.
16. Raise the side rail, and lower the bed to its lowest horizontal position.
17. Make sure the patient is comfortable and the signal light is within reach.
18. Open the privacy curtain.
19. Dispose of the disposable supplies and dirty linen following facility policy.
20. Remove and dispose of your gloves. Wash your hands.
21. Report to the nurse that you have given daily catheter care and any unusual observations.

PROCEDURE: EMPTYING A URINARY DRAINAGE BAG

1. Wash your hands.
2. Check the patient's identification bracelet and speak the patient's name.
3. Explain to the patient what you are going to do.
4. Follow facility policy for asking visitors to leave the room.
5. Collect the following equipment: a calibrated graduate, disposable gloves, and antiseptic swab.
6. Close the privacy curtain.
7. Put on the disposable gloves.

8. With the graduate positioned beneath the urinary drainage bag drain valve, open the valve and let the urine run out into the graduate.
9. After all urine has drained out, close the valve and wipe it with the antiseptic swab. Dispose of the swab.
10. Measure the urine output and record it properly on the intake and output record sheet.
11. Pour the urine into the toilet. Wash the graduate properly and put it away.
12. Remove the gloves and dispose of properly.
13. Open the privacy curtain.
14. Wash your hands.
15. Report to the nurse that you have emptied the drainage bag and any unusual observations.

General Rules for Collecting Urine Specimens

- Always wash your hands carefully before and after the procedure. It is recommended that you wear disposable gloves.
- Be careful to use the correct container, the correct method of collection, and the correct label for the specimen following facility policy.
- Be accurate in collecting specimens at the ordered times.
- When handling the container, be careful not to touch the inside of the container or lid.
- Ask the patient not to defecate or drop toilet tissue into the specimen collection.
- As always when dealing with the patient's bodily functions, be sensitive to the patient's feelings and potential embarrassment.

■ Do not allow the urine specimen to stand at room temperature for more than 30 minutes before sending it to the laboratory.

PROCEDURE: COLLECTING A ROUTINE URINE SPECIMEN

1. Wash your hands.
2. Check the patient's identification bracelet and speak the patient's name.
3. Explain to the patient what you are going to do. Allow the patient to collect the specimen if able.
4. Follow facility policy for asking visitors to leave the room.
5. Collect the following equipment: bedpan with cover (or urinal or specimen tray), specimen container with lid, calibrated graduate, label and pen, disposable bag, and disposable gloves.
6. Prepare the specimen label with information from the patient's identification bracelet.
7. Close the privacy curtain.
8. Remind the patient not to defecate into the bedpan or specimen tray and to put toilet tissue into the disposable bag.
9. Give the patient the bedpan or urinal and assist as needed (see preceding procedures).
10. Carry the bedpan or urinal to the bathroom. Measure the urine if the patient's intake and output are being recorded. Record the amount on the intake and output record sheet.
11. Pour urine into the specimen container until it is about three-fourths full. Pour the remaining urine into the toilet.

12. Put the lid and label on the container.
13. Clean and rinse the bedpan and graduate and put them in their proper places.
14. Assist the patient in washing hands.
15. Make sure the patient is comfortable and can reach the signal light.
16. Open the privacy curtain.
17. Remove and dispose of your gloves. Wash your hands.
18. Follow facility policy to take or send the urine sample to the laboratory.
19. Report to the nurse that you have taken the routine urine specimen and any unusual observations.

PROCEDURE: COLLECTING A URINE SPECIMEN FROM A CHILD OR INFANT

1. Wash your hands.
2. Check the child's identification bracelet.
3. Explain to the parents and the child what you are going to do.
4. Follow facility policy for asking visitors other than the parents to leave the room.
5. Collect the following equipment: disposable collection bag, specimen container with lid, calibrated graduate, wash basin with cotton balls, bath blanket, label and pen, and disposable gloves.
6. Prepare the specimen label with information from the patient's identification bracelet.
7. Close the privacy curtain. Lower the side rail.
8. Remove the child's diaper. Clean the perineal area with cotton balls. Dry the area carefully.

9. Remove the backing from the urine collector bag.
10. With the child lying on the back with legs parted, position the collector bag around the penis of a boy or over the perineal area of a girl, being careful not to cover the rectal area. Check that the adhesive around the bag's opening is holding to the skin.
11. Put the diaper back on. Raise the side rail.
12. If appropriate, raise the head of the bed or crib to help the urine flow to the bottom of the bag.
13. Return to the room every 30 to 60 minutes and open the diaper to see if the child has urinated.
14. Lower the side rail. Carefully remove the collector bag.
15. Wash the perineal area and dry the area well. Put the diaper back on. Raise the side rail. Lower the bed or crib to its lowest horizontal position.
16. Carry the collector bag to the bathroom. Measure the urine if the patient's intake and output are being recorded. Record the amount on the intake and output record sheet.
17. Pour urine into the specimen container. Pour any excess amount into the toilet. Dispose of the collector bag properly.
18. Put the lid and label on the container.
19. Clean and rinse the graduate and put it in the proper place.
20. Make sure the child is comfortable.
21. Open the privacy curtain.
22. Remove and dispose of your gloves. Wash your hands.

23. Follow facility policy to take or send the urine sample to the laboratory.
24. Report to the nurse that you have collected the urine specimen and any unusual observations.

PROCEDURE: COLLECTING A CLEAN-CATCH URINE SPECIMEN

1. Wash your hands.
2. Check the patient's identification bracelet and speak the patient's name.
3. Explain to the patient what you are going to do and what the patient will need to do. Allow the patient to collect the specimen alone if able.
4. Follow facility policy for asking visitors to leave the room.
5. Collect the following equipment: bedpan with cover or urinal, disposable clean-catch specimen collection kit, calibrated graduate, label and pen, and disposable gloves.
6. Prepare the specimen label with information from the patient's identification bracelet.
7. Close the privacy curtain.
8. Give the bedpan or urinal, or help the patient into the bathroom.
9. Open the collection kit. Put the lid of the specimen container upside down on a clean surface. Put on disposable gloves.
10. Using the disposable towelettes, clean the patient's perineal area (see Chapter 7). With uncircumcised males, retract the foreskin to clean the penis, and keep the foreskin retracted during the specimen collection.

11. Have the patient start urinating into the bedpan, toilet, or urinal. After the flow starts, tell the patient to stop the stream, hold the container in place, and then start urinating again. Have the patient stop again and remove the container after the sample is collected, and then let the patient finish.
12. If the container has separating parts, remove upper part of container before putting on lid. Be careful not to touch the inside of the lid when putting it on the specimen container. Place the label on the container.
13. Carry the bedpan or urinal to the bathroom. Measure the excess urine if the patient's intake and output are being recorded. Record the total amount on the intake and output record sheet.
14. Dispose of disposable equipment.
15. Clean and rinse the bedpan or urinal and graduate and put them in their proper places.
16. Assist the patient in washing hands and cleaning the perineal area if needed.
17. Make sure the patient is comfortable and can reach the signal light.
18. Open the privacy curtain. Lower the bed to the lowest horizontal position. Raise the side rail if appropriate.
19. Remove and dispose of your gloves. Wash your hands.
20. Follow facility policy to take or send the urine sample to the laboratory.
21. Report to the nurse that you have taken the clean-catch urine specimen and any unusual observations.

PROCEDURE: COLLECTING A 24-HOUR URINE SPECIMEN

1. Wash your hands.
2. Check the patient's identification bracelet and speak the patient's name.
3. Explain to the patient that all urine for a 24-hour period will be collected and preserved in a container in the bathroom.
4. Follow facility policy for asking visitors to leave the room.
5. Collect the following equipment: large urine collection container, funnel for mouth of container, bedpan with cover or urinal, ice bucket into which the urine collection container fits, calibrated graduate, labels and pen, and disposable gloves. (Some facilities may use a chemical preservative instead of ice.)
6. Prepare the specimen label with information from the patient's identification bracelet. Put the label on the container.
7. Put a label over the patient's bed that indicates the patient is on a 24-hour urine specimen.
8. Close the privacy curtain.
9. Give the bedpan or urinal, or help the patient onto the commode or into the bathroom.
10. Have the patient urinate as usual. Measure and record the urine amount if the patient is on a intake and output record. Dispose of this urine. Record this as the beginning time for the 24-hour specimen.

11. Explain to the patient the procedure for urination for the 24 hours. Do not put toilet tissue in the bedpan or urinal. The patient should use the signal light with each urination, and all urine is to be emptied into the large container. Measure and record the patient's urine output if intake and output are being recorded.
12. The bucket around the container must be kept full of ice. Staff on the next shifts should be informed to maintain the patient on the 24-hour specimen.
13. After each use clean and rinse the bedpan or urinal, the funnel, and graduate and put them in their proper places.
14. Assist the patient in washing hands and the perineal area as needed.
15. Make sure the patient is comfortable and can reach the signal light.
16. Open the privacy curtain. Lower the bed to the lowest horizontal position. Raise the side rail if appropriate.
17. After 24 hours, ask the patient to urinate again, and add this amount to the container as the end of the specimen.
18. Dispose of disposable equipment properly, and clean and put away other equipment.
19. Remove the 24-hour specimen label from above the bed.
20. Remove and dispose of your gloves. Wash your hands.
21. Follow facility policy to take or send the urine sample to the laboratory.

22. Report to the nurse that you have completed the 24-hour urine specimen and any unusual observations.

PROCEDURE: COLLECTING A DOUBLE-VOIDED URINE SPECIMEN

Note: This specimen is also called a fresh-fractional urine specimen.

1. Wash your hands.
2. Check the patient's identification bracelet and speak the patient's name.
3. Explain that because a sample of fresh urine is needed, the patient will need to urinate now and then again in 30 minutes.
4. Follow facility policy for asking visitors to leave the room.
5. Collect the following equipment: bedpan with cover (or urinal or specimen tray), specimen container with lid, calibrated graduate, label and pen, and disposable gloves.
6. Prepare the specimen label with information from the patient's identification bracelet.
7. Close the privacy curtain.
8. Give the patient the bedpan or urinal and assist as needed (see preceding procedures). Put on the disposable gloves. Ask the patient to urinate fully.
9. Carry the bedpan or urinal to the bathroom. Measure the urine if the patient's intake and output are being recorded. Record the amount on the intake and output record sheet. Then discard this urine.

10. Clean and rinse the bedpan and graduate and put them in their proper places.
11. Assist the patient in washing the hands and the perineal area if needed.
12. Remove and dispose of your gloves.
13. Make sure the patient is comfortable and can reach the signal light.
14. Open the privacy curtain.
15. Wash your hands.
16. In about 30 minutes return to the patient and explain that the for a fresh sample you need the patient to urinate again. Remind the patient not to defecate or put toilet tissue in the bedpan.
17. Close the privacy curtain.
18. Give the patient the bedpan or urinal and assist as needed. Put on the disposable gloves.
19. Carry the bedpan or urinal to the bathroom. Measure the urine if the patient's intake and output are being recorded. Record the amount on the intake and output record sheet.
20. Pour the urine into the specimen collection container. Put the lid and label on the container. Discard any urine remaining.
21. Clean and rinse the bedpan and graduate and put them in their proper places.
22. Assist the patient in washing the hands and perineal area if needed. Remove and dispose of your gloves.
23. Make sure the patient is comfortable and can reach the signal light.
24. Open the privacy curtain.
25. Wash your hands.

26. Follow facility policy to take or send the urine sample to the laboratory. Or if instructed, perform one of the following urine tests with this sample yourself.
27. Report to the nurse that you have taken the double-voided urine specimen and any unusual observations.

PROCEDURE: PERFORMING THE TESTAPE URINE TEST

1. Wash your hands.
2. Check the patient's identification bracelet and speak the patient's name.
3. Explain to the patient what you are going to do.
4. Follow facility policy for asking visitors to leave the room.
5. Obtain a Testape dispenser with color chart and disposable gloves.
6. Close the privacy curtain.
7. Collect a urine specimen (see preceding procedure), wearing the disposable gloves.
8. Remove about 1.5 inches of Testape from the dispenser.
9. Dip one end of the Testape into the urine specimen and withdraw it.
10. Holding the tape vertical with the wet end down, use your wristwatch to time 60 seconds.
11. Hold the Testape next to the color chart on the dispenser and match its color with the color on the chart. Read the number of that color.
12. Carefully dispose of the used Testape and the urine sample.

13. Remove the disposable gloves. Wash your hands.
14. Open the privacy curtain.
15. Report to the nurse the number from the color chart and any unusual observations.

PROCEDURE: PERFORMING THE CLINITEST URINE TEST

1. Wash your hands.
2. Check the patient's identification bracelet and speak the patient's name.
3. Explain to the patient what you are going to do.
4. Follow facility policy for asking visitors to leave the room.
5. Collect the following equipment: Clinitest kit (with test tube, medicine dropper, Clinitest tablets, test tube holder, and color chart), paper towels, disposable gloves, and paper cup of water.
6. Close the privacy curtain.
7. Collect a urine specimen (see earlier procedure), wearing the disposable gloves.
8. Put paper towels on the working area.
9. Rinse the medicine dropper in the paper cup of water.
10. With the test tube upright in the holder, put 5 drops of urine in the test tube.
11. Rinse the dropper in the paper cup.
12. Put 10 drops of clean water into the test tube.
13. Remove one Clinitest tablet from the bottle by carefully pouring one tablet from the bottle into the bottle cap--do not touch the tablet.

14. Pour the tablet from the bottle cap into the test tube and recap the bottle tightly.
15. Watch until the boiling reaction has stopped in the test tube; using your wrist watch, wait an additional 15 seconds and gently shake the test tube.
16. Put the color chart next to the test tube and match the color of the liquid with the appropriate color on the chart. Read the number for that color.
17. Carefully dispose of the liquid from the test tube and the remainder of the urine sample and rinse cup. Wash and rinse the medicine dropper and the test tube.
18. Clean up the area and dispose of the paper towels covering the surface.
19. Remove the disposable gloves. Wash your hands.
20. Open the privacy curtain.
21. Report to the nurse the number from the color chart and any unusual observations.

PROCEDURE: PERFORMING THE ACETEST URINE TEST

1. Wash your hands.
2. Check the patient's identification bracelet and speak the patient's name.
3. Explain to the patient what you are going to do.
4. Follow facility policy for asking visitors to leave the room.

5. Collect the following equipment: Acetest tablets and color chart, medicine dropper, paper towels, disposable gloves, and paper cup of water.
6. Close the privacy curtain.
7. Collect a urine specimen (see earlier procedure), wearing the disposable gloves.
8. Put paper towels on the working surface area.
9. Remove one Acetest tablet from the bottle by carefully pouring one tablet from the bottle into the bottle cap--do not touch the tablet.
10. Pour the tablet from the bottle cap onto the paper towel and recap the bottle tightly.
11. Rinse the medicine dropper in the paper cup of water.
12. Draw some urine from the sample into the medicine dropper.
13. Drop one drop of urine onto the Acetest tablet.
14. Using your wristwatch, wait for 30 seconds.
15. Put the color chart next to the tablet and match the color of the tablet with the appropriate color on the chart. Read the result for that color.
16. Carefully dispose of the used tablet and the remainder of the urine sample and rinse cup. Wash and rinse the medicine dropper and the test tube.
17. Clean up the area and dispose of the paper towels covering the surface.
18. Remove the disposable gloves. Wash your hands.
19. Open the privacy curtain.
20. Report to the nurse the result from the color chart and any unusual observations.

PROCEDURE: PERFORMING THE KETOSTIX URINE TEST

1. Wash your hands.
2. Check the patient's identification bracelet and speak the patient's name.
3. Explain to the patient what you are going to do.
4. Follow facility policy for asking visitors to leave the room.
5. Obtain a Ketostix strip dispenser with color chart and disposable gloves.
6. Close the privacy curtain.
7. Collect a urine specimen (see earlier procedure), wearing the disposable gloves.
8. Remove one strip from the dispenser and recap the bottle tightly.
9. Dip the strip test area completely into the urine specimen and withdraw it, letting it drip back into the specimen.
10. Use your wristwatch to time 15 seconds.
11. Hold the strip next to the color chart on the dispenser bottle and match its color with the color on the chart to determine the result.
12. Carefully dispose of the used strip and the urine sample. Clean and put away equipment.
13. Remove the disposable gloves. Wash your hands.
14. Open the privacy curtain.
15. Report to the nurse the result from the color chart and any unusual observations.

PROCEDURE: PERFORMING URINE STRAINING

1. Wash your hands.
2. Check the patient's identification bracelet and speak the patient's name.
3. Explain to the patient what you are going to do.
4. Follow facility policy for asking visitors to leave the room.
5. Gather the following equipment: disposable paper strainer or gauze square, specimen container and label, bedpan or urinal, and disposable gloves.
6. Close the privacy curtain.
7. Collect a urine specimen (see earlier procedure), wearing the disposable gloves.
8. Put the disposable paper strainer or gauze square into the specimen container and pour the urine through it.
9. Unless the urine is needed for a specimen, dispose of it appropriately and examine the stainer or gauze carefully.
10. If you see any particles or crystals in the strainer or gauze, put it in the specimen container and label the container with the patient information, date, and time.
11. Clean and put away equipment.
12. Remove the disposable gloves. Wash your hands.
13. Open the privacy curtain.
14. Follow facility policy to take or send the specimen to the laboratory.
15. Report to the nurse the result of the straining and any unusual observations.

General Rules for Bowel Elimination

- For patients who cannot leave the bed easily to reach the bathroom a bedpan is generally used for bowel movements.
- Offer the patient the bedpan periodically when providing care, and always bring it as soon as requested.
- Be sure the bedpan is warm before offering it.
- Raise the head of the bed as high as possible.
- Give the patient privacy, or stay nearby if the patient may need assistance.
- Always give the patient sufficient time for a bowel movement; never rush the patient.
- After a bowel movement, cover the bedpan and take it to the bathroom immediately after use; collect a specimen carefully if ordered (see later procedure).
- Assist the patient with perineal care if needed (see Chapter 7).
- It is generally recommended that you wear disposable gloves when handling fecal material.

General Rules for Giving an Enema

- An enema may be given to promote complete emptying of the patient's lower bowel or to cleanse the bowel in preparation for a medical procedure.
- Be careful and exact in the amount of solution to use in an enema, usually not more than 500 ml for children or 1000 ml for an adult.
- Be careful not to insert the enema tube more than 2 to 4 inches into the rectum for an adult or the intestine may be injured.

- Since an enema may be dangerous for some patients, administer an enema only when clearly ordered to do so.
- As with all procedures involving urinary or bowel elimination, be sensitive to the patient's feelings and likely embarrassment or discomfort.
- Never administer more than three enemas at one time to a patient.

PROCEDURE: GIVING A CLEANSING ENEMA

1. Wash your hands.
2. Check the patient's identification bracelet and speak the patient's name.
3. Explain to the patient what you are going to do.
4. Follow facility policy for asking visitors to leave the room.
5. Collect the following equipment: disposable enema kit (container, tubing, and clamp), graduated pitcher, lubricant, bath thermometer, bed protector, paper towels, toilet tissue, bath blanket, bedpan and cover, disposable gloves, and the ordered enema solution (enema soap or salt).
6. Close the privacy curtain.
7. Raise the bed to a high level to ease your body movements. Lower the side rail.
8. Put the bath blanket over the patient to prevent exposure, and fanfold the top bed linen to the foot of the bed.
9. Put the bed protector under the patient's buttocks and the bedpan at the foot of the bed.

10. Raise the side rail while you prepare the solution in the bathroom.
11. Close the clamp on the enema tubing.
12. Adjust the water temperature to 105 degrees F (40.5 degrees C). Use the graduated pitcher to measure the ordered amount (often 1000 ml for adults) and mix in the ordered solution (such as one premixed package of soap or 2 teaspoons of salt). Pour the liquid into the enema bag.
13. Let a little of the solution flow through the tubing to remove air, and then clamp the tube closed.
14. Lower the headrest and the side rail and position the patient on the left side with right knee forward (left Sims' position). Drape the bath blanket so that only the anal area is exposed.
15. Put on the disposable gloves.
16. Lubricate the tubing thoroughly for 2 to 4 inches from the tip.
17. Expose the anal area by raising the upper buttock with one hand, while the other hand handles the tubing.
18. Ask the patient to take deep slow breaths through the mouth while you gently insert the tip of the tubing 2 to 4 inches into the rectum. Do not keep pushing if you feel resistance or the patient complains of pain.
19. Open the clamp on the tubing and raise the bag about 12 inches above the anus (18 inches above the mattress).
20. Ask the patient to keep breathing slowly.

21. Allow the solution to flow slowly through the tube unless the patient feels an urge to defecate or cramps, or the solution leaks out. If one of these occurs, close the clamp for a moment.
22. When the bag is empty or nearly so, close the clamp and slowly withdraw the tube. Wrap the tube in paper towels and put it inside the enema container bag.
23. Encourage the patient to retain the enema solution for at least 5 minutes. Help the patient to the bathroom or to use the bedpan (see earlier procedure). Ask the patient not to flush the toilet. Leave the patient alone if safe, or check on the patient if necessary.
24. Dispose of the enema equipment.
25. When the patient has finished the bowel movement, inspect the stool and obtain a specimen if ordered see later procedure). Ask the nurse to examine the stool if it looks unusual in any way.
26. Help the patient with perineal cleaning if necessary.
27. Empty, clean, and put away the bedpan and any other equipment.
28. Remove the disposable gloves.
29. Remove the bed protector. Fold the bed linen back into place and remove the bath blanket.
30. Help the patient wash the hands if necessary.
31. Raise the side rail. Lower the bed to its lowest horizontal position.
32. Make sure the patient is comfortable and can reach the signal light.
33. Open the privacy curtain.
34. Dispose of dirty laundry.

35. Wash your hands.
36. Report to the nurse that you have given the enema, the appearance of the stool, and any unusual observations.

PROCEDURE: GIVING A COMMERCIAL ENEMA

1. Wash your hands.
2. Check the patient's identification bracelet and speak the patient's name.
3. Explain to the patient what you are going to do.
4. Follow facility policy for asking visitors to leave the room.
5. Collect the following equipment: commercially prepared enema (plastic squeeze bottle containing solution and prelubricated tip), bed protector, toilet tissue, bath blanket, bedpan and cover, and disposable gloves.
6. Close the privacy curtain.
7. Raise the bed to a high level to ease your body movements. Lower the side rail.
8. Put the bath blanket over the patient to prevent exposure, and fanfold the top bed linen to the foot of the bed.
9. Put the bed protector under the patient's buttocks and the bedpan at the foot of the bed.
10. Lower the headrest and position the patient on the left side with right knee forward (left Sims' position). Drape the bath blanket so that only the anal area is exposed.
11. Put on the disposable gloves.

12. Open the enema package and remove the cap to expose the prelubricated tip. (If ordered, warm the enema bottle in warm water using a bath thermometer.)
13. Expose the anal area by raising the upper buttock with one hand, while the other hand handles the enema.
14. Ask the patient to take deep slow breaths through the mouth while you gently insert the tip 2 inches into the rectum. Do not keep pushing if you feel resistance or the patient complains of pain.
15. Ask the patient to keep breathing slowly.
16. Slowly squeeze the bottle and roll up the empty part from the bottom--do not release pressure on the bottle while giving the enema.
17. Continue until the bottle is empty unless the patient feels an urge to defecate or cramps, or the solution leaks out. If one of these occurs, stop squeezing momentarily but do not release pressure on the squeeze bottle.
18. When the bottle is empty, slowly withdraw the tip. Put the empty bottle back in the original packaging for disposal.
19. Help the patient to the bathroom or to use the bedpan (see earlier procedure). Ask the patient not to flush the toilet. Leave the patient alone if safe, or check on the patient if necessary.
20. Dispose of the used enema container.
21. When the patient has finished the bowel movement, inspect the stool and obtain a specimen if ordered. Ask the nurse to examine the stool if it looks unusual in any way.

22. Help the patient with perineal cleaning if necessary.
23. Empty, clean, and put away the bedpan and any other equipment.
24. Remove the disposable gloves.
25. Remove the bed protector. Fold the bed linen back into place and remove the bath blanket.
26. Help the patient wash the hands if necessary.
27. Raise the side rail. Lower the bed to its lowest horizontal position.
28. Make sure the patient is comfortable and can reach the signal light.
29. Open the privacy curtain.
30. Dispose of dirty laundry.
31. Wash your hands.
32. Report to the nurse that you have given the enema, the appearance of the stool, and any unusual observations.

PROCEDURE: GIVING AN OIL RETENTION ENEMA

1. Wash your hands.
2. Check the patient's identification bracelet and speak the patient's name.
3. Explain to the patient what you are going to do.
4. Follow facility policy for asking visitors to leave the room.
5. Collect the following equipment: prepared oil retention enema kit (plastic squeeze bottle containing solution and prelubricated tip), bed protector, toilet tissue, bath blanket, bedpan and cover, and disposable gloves.
6. Close the privacy curtain.

7. Raise the bed to a high level to ease your body movements. Lower the side rail.
8. Put the bath blanket over the patient to prevent exposure, and fanfold the top bed linen to the foot of the bed.
9. Put the bed protector under the patient's buttocks and the bedpan at the foot of the bed.
10. Lower the headrest and position the patient on the left side with right knee forward (left Sims' position). Drape the bath blanket so that only the anal area is exposed.
11. Put on the disposable gloves.
12. Open the oil retention enema package and remove the cap to expose the prelubricated tip. (If ordered, warm the enema in warm water using a bath thermometer.)
13. Expose the anal area by raising the upper buttock with one hand, while the other hand handles the enema.
14. Ask the patient to take deep slow breaths through the mouth while you gently insert the tip 2 inches into the rectum. Do not keep pushing if you feel resistance or the patient complains of pain.
15. Ask the patient to keep breathing slowly.
16. Slowly squeeze the bottle--do not release pressure on the bottle while giving the enema.
17. Continue until the bottle is empty unless the patient feels an urge to defecate or cramps, or the solution leaks out. If one of these occurs, stop squeezing momentarily but do not release pressure on the squeeze bottle.

18. When the bottle is empty, slowly withdraw the tip. Put the empty bottle back in the original packaging for disposal.
19. Remove the disposable gloves.
20. Tell the patient the enema solution must be retained for the length of time ordered (usually 20 minutes). Leave the patient in the same position, if possible. If you leave the patient during this time, be sure the signal light is within reach and the side rail is up; check frequently on the patient.
21. You may be ordered to give a soap cleansing enema following the oil retention enema (see earlier procedure).
22. Help the patient to the bathroom or to use the bedpan (see earlier procedure). Ask the patient not to flush the toilet. Leave the patient alone if safe, or check on the patient if necessary.
23. Dispose of the used enema container.
24. When the patient has finished the bowel movement, inspect the stool and obtain a specimen if ordered. Ask the nurse to examine the stool if it looks unusual in any way.
25. Help the patient with perineal cleaning if necessary.
26. Empty, clean, and put away the bedpan and any other equipment.
27. Remove the bed protector. Fold the bed linen back into place and remove the bath blanket.
28. Help the patient wash the hands if necessary.
29. Raise the side rail. Lower the bed to its lowest horizontal position.

30. Make sure the patient is comfortable and can reach the signal light.
31. Open the privacy curtain.
32. Dispose of dirty laundry.
33. Wash your hands.
34. Report to the nurse that you have given the oil retention enema, the appearance of the stool, and any unusual observations.

PROCEDURE: RECTAL TUBE USE

1. Wash your hands.
2. Check the patient's identification bracelet and speak the patient's name.
3. Explain to the patient what you are going to do and that the rectal tube will help relieve gas.
4. Follow facility policy for asking visitors to leave the room.
5. Collect the following equipment: disposable rectal tube with bag, lubricant, bath blanket, adhesive tape, and disposable gloves.
6. Close the privacy curtain.
7. Raise the bed to a high level to ease your body movements. Lower the side rail.
8. Put the bath blanket over the patient to prevent exposure, and fanfold the top bed linen to the foot of the bed.
9. Lower the headrest and position the patient on the left side with right knee forward (left Sims' position). Drape the bath blanket so that only the anal area is exposed.
10. Put on the disposable gloves.
11. Lubricate 2 to 4 inches of the tubing.

12. Expose the anal area by raising the upper buttock with one hand, while the other hand handles the tubing.

13. Ask the patient to take deep slow breaths through the mouth while you gently insert the tip 2 inches into the rectum. Do not keep pushing if you feel resistance or the patient complains of pain.

14. Tape the tube to the patient's buttocks to keep it in place.

15. Leave the tube in place for the ordered amount of time (usually 20 minutes). If you leave the patient, raise the side rail, lower the bed, and be sure the signal light is within reach. Remove the gloves and wash your hands.

16. Return to the patient, raise the bed, and lower the side rail.

17. Put on disposable gloves.

18. Remove the tube slowly and gently. Dispose of the tubing and flatus bag. Ask the patient whether gas was expelled.

19. Fold the bed linen back into place and remove the bath blanket.

20. Raise the side rail. Lower the bed to its lowest horizontal position.

21. Make sure the patient is comfortable and can reach the signal light.

22. Open the privacy curtain.

23. Wash your hands.

24. Report to the nurse that you have inserted and removed the rectal tube, the appearance of any stool passed into the flatus bag, the patient's comments about expelling gas, and any unusual observations.

PROCEDURE: INSERTING A RECTAL SUPPOSITORY

1. Wash your hands.
2. Check the patient's identification bracelet and speak the patient's name.
3. Explain to the patient what you are going to do and why the rectal suppository was ordered (to help elimination, relieve pain, or other medical purpose).
4. Follow facility policy for asking visitors to leave the room.
5. Collect the following equipment: rectal suppository, lubricant, bath blanket, bedpan, and disposable gloves.
6. Close the privacy curtain.
7. Raise the bed to a high level to ease your body movements. Lower the side rail.
8. Put the bath blanket over the patient to prevent exposure, and fanfold the top bed linen to the foot of the bed.
9. Lower the headrest and position the patient on the left side with right knee forward (left Sims' position). Drape the bath blanket so that only the anal area is exposed.
10. Put on the disposable gloves.
11. Lubricate the suppository over all its surface.
12. Expose the anal area by raising the upper buttock with one hand, while the other hand handles the suppository.
13. Ask the patient to take deep slow breaths through the mouth while you gently insert the suppository into the rectum. Slide it along one side of the rectum about as far as your index finger can push it (2 inches). Do not keep

pushing if you feel resistance or the patient complains of pain.
14. Remove the gloves and wash your hands.
15. Fold the bed linen back into place and remove the bath blanket. Put the bedpan nearby and ask the patient to signal you when needed for bowel elimination.
16. If you leave the patient, raise the side rail, lower the bed, and be sure the signal light is within reach. Check on the patient frequently.
17. Give the patient the bedpan when needed (see earlier procedure).
18. Open the privacy curtain.
19. Report to the nurse that you have inserted the rectal suppository, the patient's response to it, and any unusual observations.

PROCEDURE: COLLECTING A STOOL SPECIMEN

1. Tell the patient you need to collect a stool specimen and ask the patient to signal you before having a bowel movement.
2. Have ready the following equipment: bedpan and cover or specimen pan for bathroom toilet, specimen container, label and pen, tongue depressor, toilet tissue and disposable bag, and disposable gloves.
3. Go to the patient when signaled for a bowel movement.
4. Wash your hands.
5. Check the patient's identification bracelet and speak the patient's name. Complete the specimen label with the patient's information.

6. Follow facility policy for asking visitors to leave the room.
7. Close the privacy curtain.
8. Give the bedpan to the patient (see earlier procedure) or put the specimen pan in the bathroom toilet.
9. Ask the patient to urinate in the urinal rather than the bedpan and not to put toilet tissue in the bedpan (provide the disposable bag for tissue).
10. Make sure the patient can reach the signal light.
11. Tell the patient to signal for assistance or when finished.
12. Wash your hands.
13. Leave the room and close the door.
14. After the patient signals, return to the room.
15. Wash your hands and put on disposable gloves.
16. Cover and take the bedpan or specimen pan to the bathroom.
17. Use the tongue depressor to transfer about 2 tablespoons of feces from the bedpan or specimen pan to the specimen container. Put the lid on the container without touching the inside of the container or lid.
18. Use the disposable bag to dispose of the tongue depressor and used tissue.
19. Empty the bedpan into the toilet, and clean and put it away.
20. Remove the gloves and dispose of them.
21. Open the privacy curtain.
22. Make sure the patient is comfortable and can reach the signal light.
23. Wash your hands.

24. Follow facility policy to take or send the stool specimen to laboratory.
25. Report to the nurse that you have collected the stool specimen and any unusual observations.

General Rules for Ostomy Care

- Because the patient with an ostomy may feel angry, depressed, helpless, or a range of other emotions, be especially sensitive when providing care.
- Report significant behavior or emotional changes to the nurse.
- Skin care around the ostomy site is an important consideration for these patients. Report any sign of skin breakdown.
- Patients who are able to should be allowed to manage the ostomy by themselves or to assist.
- Change of the ostomy bag whenever soiled and the use of deodorants will help prevent odors and make the patient more comfortable.
- Ostomy drainage should always be recorded and reported to the nurse.

PROCEDURE: OSTOMY CARE

1. Wash your hands.
2. Check the patient's identification bracelet and speak the patient's name.
3. Explain to the patient what you are going to do and what the patient can do to help.
4. Follow facility policy for asking visitors to leave the room.

5. Collect the following equipment: bedpan and cover, bed protector, bath blanket, wash basin, bath thermometer, the appropriate soap, disposable gloves, disposable bag, paper towels, toilet tissue, clean ostomy belt, and clean stoma bag (also called an ostomy appliance).
6. Close the privacy curtain.
7. Raise the bed to a high level to ease your body movements. Lower the side rail.
8. Put the bath blanket over the patient and fold the top bed linens to the foot of the bed.
9. Put the bed protector under the patient's hips and buttocks.
10. Prepare the basin of wash water at 105 degrees F (46 degrees C).
11. Put on disposable gloves.
12. Disconnect the used stoma bag from the ostomy belt and open and remove the belt.
13. Carefully remove the stoma bag from the patient's skin and put it in the bedpan.
14. With toilet tissue carefully wipe around the opening in the skin (stoma) and put the tissue in the bedpan. Cover the bedpan.
15. Gently wash the skin around the stoma, using soap as ordered. Rinse and dry. Use lubricant around the stoma as ordered.
16. Put the new ostomy belt around the patient and attach the clean stoma bag.
17. Put the stoma bag in place on the skin, peeling off the backing of the adhesive surface.
18. Remove the bed protector. Fold the top bed linen back up and remove the bath blanket.

19. Raise the side rail. Lower the bed to its lowest horizontal position.
20. Make sure the patient is comfortable and can reach the signal light.
21. Take the bedpan to the bathroom and empty the stoma bag into the toilet. Put the empty bag in the disposable bag.
22. Dispose of the disposable bag and used paper towels and tissues.
23. Wash the bedpan and wash basin and put them away.
24. Remove and dispose of the gloves. Wash your hands.
25. Open the privacy curtain.
26. Report to the nurse that you have given ostomy care and any unusual observations.

Chapter 12
Applying Heat and Cold

This chapter includes information on the following:
Principles of heat and cold applications
General rules for heat applications
Procedure: Giving a hot soak
Procedure: Giving a sitz bath
Procedure: Applying a hot water bottle
Procedure: Applying a hot compress
Procedure: Applying a commercial hot compress
Procedure: Applying an electric (aquamatic) heat pad
Procedure: Using a heat lamp
General rules for cold applications
Procedure: Giving a cooling sponge bath
Procedure: Applying a cold compress
Procedure: Giving a cold soak
Procedure: Applying an ice bag
Procedure: Applying a disposable cold pack

Principles of Heat and Cold Applications

- ▶ Heat applications may be prescribed to improve circulation, reduce pain, or ease joint movement.
- ▶ Cold applications are prescribed to reduce a fever or to slow circulation in order to reduce swelling and pain or to control bleeding.
- ▶ Be exact in the body location for a hot or cold application, the temperature of the application, and the length of time.

- Check the patient frequently throughout the application to check the application temperature and the patient's response.
- Take care to prevent accidents, and follow safety guidelines when working with electrical equipment, particularly around water.
- Observe the patient's skin under the application and immediately report any discolored areas.
- When using bottles or containers with a cap or stopper, be sure the cap or stopper does not contact the patient's skin because its temperature is more extreme than rest of the bottle or container. Check the container carefully for leaks before using.

General Rules for Heat Applications

- Always use a bath thermometer to check the temperature of hot moist applications.
- Never use equipment for heat applications unless you are completely familiar with it.
- Always use the temperature instructed for the patient. Pay special attention with elderly patients, infants, and others more susceptible to burns.
- Always carefully time the heat application and never exceed the instructed length.
- Monitor the patient carefully and immediately report any signs of problems or patient complaints of pain or burning.
- Explain to the patient the purpose of the heat application and the risks; do not let the patient change the temperature level or length of the application.

PROCEDURE: GIVING A HOT SOAK

1. Wash your hands.
2. Check the patient's identification bracelet and speak the patient's name.
3. Explain to the patient that you are going to give a hot soak.
4. Follow facility policy for asking visitors to leave the room.
5. Collect the following equipment: wash basin or a foot or arm basin, bath thermometer, bath blanket, towels, and waterproof bed protector.
6. Close the privacy curtain.
7. Raise the bed to a high level to ease your body movements. Help the patient assume a comfortable position.
8. Place a waterproof bed protector under the body area to be treated.
9. Fill the basin halfway with 105 degree F water (40.5 degrees C), using the bath thermometer.
10. Expose the area to be treated.
11. Slowly place the hand, foot, or arm into the basin, noting the time the treatment begins.
12. Cover the patient with the bath blanket.
13. Every 5 minutes, check the water temperature. When you change the water, keep the body area warm by wrapping it in a towel.
14. Every 5 minutes, check the area being treated for redness. If the patient is feeling any pain or discomfort, remove the area from the water and wrap it in a towel. Report the problem to the nurse immediately.
15. When the treatment is complete, remove the extremity from the water and dry it with a towel. Remove the bath blanket.

16. Lower the bed to a safe and comfortable position.
17. Make sure the side rails are raised and the patient can reach the signal light.
18. Open the privacy curtain.
19. Clean and return equipment to its proper location.
20. Place soiled linens in the laundry bag.
21. Wash your hands.
22. Report to the nurse that you have give the patient a hot soak and how well the procedure was tolerated.

PROCEDURE: GIVING A SITZ BATH

1. Wash your hands.
2. Check the patient's identification bracelet and speak the patient's name.
3. Explain to the patient that you are going to give a sitz bath.
4. Follow facility policy for asking visitors to leave the room.
5. Collect the following equipment: disposable sitz bath kit, bath thermometer, towel, two bath blankets, water pitcher, clean gown, and wheelchair (if necessary).
6. Close the privacy curtain and room door.
7. Put the sitz bath bowl into the toilet bowl, making sure the overflow spout faces the front of the toilet.
8. Help the patient put on robe and slippers.
9. Help the patient out of bed and to the bathroom, using the wheelchair if necessary (see Chapter 6 procedure).

10. Fill the pitcher with water, testing the temperature with the bath thermometer. The water should be 100 to 104 degrees F (38 to 40 degrees C) for cleaning purposes, or 105 to 110 degrees F (40.5 to 43 degrees C) for circulation improvement.
11. Fill the bowl halfway with water.
12. Close the clamp on the tubing. Fill the bag with water from the pitcher, and close the bag.
13. Hang the bag 12 inches above the bowl.
14. Help the patient remove the robe and raise the gown to the waist.
15. Help the patient sit in the sitz bath.
16. To keep the patient warm, place one bath blanket around the shoulders and the other over the legs.
17. Insert the end of the tubing into the hole in the front of the sitz bowl.
18. Open the clamp and adjust the water flow. Note the time the sitz bath begins.
19. Make sure the patient can reach the signal light.
20. Check the patient every 5 minutes. If the patient feels faint, weak, or drowsy, stop the sitz bath and return the patient to bed.
21. After the prescribed time, close the clamp and remove the tubing from the bowl.
22. Help the patient out of the sitz bath, and dry the patient's body with a towel. Help the patient put on a clean gown if necessary.
23. Help the patient return to bed.
24. Lower the bed to a safe and comfortable position.
25. Make sure the side rails are raised and the patient can reach the signal light.

26. Open the privacy curtain and door.
27. Discard all disposable equipment and trash, and place soiled linens in the laundry bag.
28. Wash your hands.
29. Report to the nurse that you have given the patient a sitz bath and how well the procedure was tolerated.

PROCEDURE: APPLYING A HOT WATER BOTTLE

1. Wash your hands.
2. Check the patient's identification bracelet and speak the patient's name.
3. Explain to the patient that you are going to give a hot water bottle treatment.
4. Follow facility policy for asking visitors to leave the room.
5. Collect the following equipment: hot water bottle, bath thermometer, pitcher, flannel cover, and paper towels.
6. Close the privacy curtain.
7. Raise the bed to a high level to ease your body movements.
8. To check the bottle for leaks, fill it with hot tap water, close it and turn it upside down. Empty the bottle.
9. Fill the pitcher with water, testing the temperature with the bath thermometer. For infants or the elderly, use 105 to 115 degree F water (40.5 to 46 degrees C), and for older children and adults use 115 to 125 degree F water (46 to 51.6 degrees C); or follow facility policy for temperature.

10. Fill the bottle two-thirds full with water from the pitcher.
11. Remove excess air from the bottle by squeezing the empty (top) part of the bottle. Fasten the stopper tightly.
12. Dry the outside of the bottle with the paper towels.
13. Place the flannel cover on the bottle.
14. Place the bottle on the prescribed body part, noting the time the treatment begins.
15. Check the skin under the bottle every 5 minutes. If redness, blisters, or swelling appear, or if the patient complains about pain or discomfort, stop the treatment and report the problem to the nurse immediately.
16. Remove the bottle after the prescribed length of treatment.
17. Lower the bed to a safe and comfortable position.
18. Make sure the side rails are raised and the patient can reach the signal light.
19. Open the privacy curtain.
20. Remove the flannel cover, and empty the bottle.
21. Clean the bottle, return equipment to its proper location, and put the flannel cover in the laundry bag.
22. Wash your hands.
23. Report to the nurse that you have given the patient a hot water bottle treatment and your observations of the patient's skin condition.

PROCEDURE: APPLYING A HOT COMPRESS

1. Wash your hands.
2. Check the patient's identification bracelet and speak the patient's name.
3. Explain to the patient that you are going to apply a hot compress.
4. Follow facility policy for asking visitors to leave the room.
5. Collect the following equipment: waterproof bed protector, basin, bath thermometer, washcloth or gauze pads, plastic wrap, bath towel, and tape or rolled gauze.
6. Close the privacy curtain.
7. Raise the bed to a high level to ease your body movements.
8. Place the waterproof bed protector under the body area to be treated. Make sure the patient is comfortable.
9. Fill the basin halfway with 110 degree F water (43 degree C), using the bath thermometer.
10. Place the washcloth or gauze pad in the basin and wring it out thoroughly.
11. Apply the compress to the proper area, noting the time.
12. Cover the compress with the plastic wrap, then cover the whole area with the bath towel.
13. To hold the towel in place, secure it with the tape or rolled gauze.
14. Make sure the patient can reach the signal light.

15. Check the treated area every 5 minutes for redness. If this appears, or if the patient complains of pain or discomfort, stop the treatment and report the problem to the nurse immediately.
16. Change the compress if it becomes cool.
17. After 20 minutes, remove the compress and dry the area with the bath towel.
18. Lower the bed to a safe and comfortable position.
19. Make sure the side rails are raised and the patient can reach the signal light.
20. Open the privacy curtain.
21. Return equipment to its proper location, and discard trash. Place soiled linens in the laundry bag.
22. Wash your hands.
23. Report to the nurse that you have applied a hot compress to the patient and your observations of the patient's skin condition.

PROCEDURE: APPLYING A COMMERCIAL HOT COMPRESS

1. Wash your hands.
2. Check the patient's identification bracelet and speak the patient's name.
3. Explain to the patient that you are going to apply a hot compress.
4. Follow facility policy for asking visitors to leave the room.
5. Collect the following equipment: a commercial compress, ultraviolet heating lamp, towel, tape or rolled gauze, and waterproof bed protector.
6. Close the privacy curtain.

7. Heat the compress under the ultraviolet heating lamp for the instructed time (usually 10 minutes).
8. Raise the bed to a high level to ease your body movements.
9. Place the waterproof bed protector under the body area to be treated. Make sure the patient is comfortable.
10. Open the compress and apply it to the proper area, noting the time.
11. Cover the compress with the towel.
12. To hold the towel in place, secure it with the tape or rolled gauze.
13. Make sure the patient can reach the signal light.
14. Check the treated area every 5 minutes for redness. If this appears, or if the patient complains of pain or discomfort, stop the treatment and report the problem to the nurse immediately.
15. Change the compress if it becomes cool.
16. After 20 minutes, remove the compress and dry the area with the towel.
17. Lower the bed to a safe and comfortable level.
18. Make sure the side rails are raised and the patient can reach the signal light.
19. Open the privacy curtain.
20. Return equipment to its proper location, and discard trash. Place soiled linens in the laundry bag.
21. Wash your hands.
22. Report to the nurse that you have applied a hot compress and your observations of the patient's skin condition.

PROCEDURE: APPLYING AN ELECTRIC (AQUAMATIC) HEAT PAD

1. Wash your hands.
2. Check the patient's identification bracelet and speak the patient's name.
3. Explain to the patient that you are going to apply a heating pad.
4. Follow facility policy for asking visitors to leave the room.
5. Collect the following equipment: aquamatic pad and heating unit, pad cover, tape or rolled gauze, and distilled water.
6. Close the privacy curtain.
7. Raise the bed to a high level to ease your body movements.
8. If the heating unit is not already prepared, fill it two-thirds with distilled water.
9. To remove air bubbles, lower the pad below the heating unit and tilt the unit from side to side.
10. If the heating unit is not preset, set the temperature at 105 degrees F (40.5 degrees C) or following facility policy.
11. Insert the pad into the cover.
12. Plug the cord into an electric outlet.
13. Place the heating unit on the bedside stand, making sure the tubing is smooth and the pad and tubing are level with the unit.
14. Apply the pad to the body area to be treated, noting the time the treatment begins.
15. To hold the pad in place, secure it with tape or rolled gauze. Never use pins.
16. Make sure the patient can reach the signal light.

17. Check the treated area every 15 to 20 minutes for redness or swelling. If these problems occur, or if the patient complains of pain or discomfort, stop the treatment and report the problem to the nurse immediately.
18. After the specified time, remove the pad and unplug the unit.
19. Lower the bed to a safe and comfortable level.
20. Make sure the side rails are raised and the patient can reach the signal light.
21. Open the privacy curtain.
22. Return equipment to its proper location.
23. Wash your hands.
24. Report to the nurse that you have applied an aquamatic pad and your observations of the patient's skin condition.

PROCEDURE: USING A HEAT LAMP

1. Wash your hands.
2. Check the patient's identification bracelet and speak the patient's name.
3. Explain to the patient that you are going to give a heat lamp treatment.
4. Follow facility policy for asking visitors to leave the room.
5. Obtain a heat lamp, bath blanket, bath towel, and tape measure. Follow facility policy to use the correct wattage bulb in the heat lamp.
6. Close the privacy curtain.
7. Raise the bed to a high level to ease your body movements.
8. Plug in the heat lamp.

9. Cover the patient with the bath blanket. Reaching under the blanket, pull down the top linens and expose only the body area to be treated.
10. Position the lamp so that it is directed at the area to be treated. Use the tape measure to make sure the lamp is at least 18 inches away from the body.
11. Note the time the treatment begins.
12. Every 5 minutes, check the treated area for redness. If this occurs, or if the patient complains of pain or discomfort, stop the treatment and report the problem to the nurse immediately.
13. After the instructed treatment time, usually not more than 15 minutes, turn off the lamp and remove it.
14. Remove the bath blanket and readjust the top linens.
15. Lower the bed to a safe and comfortable position.
16. Make sure the side rails are raised and the patient can reach the signal light.
17. Open the privacy curtain.
18. Return equipment to its proper location, and discard soiled linens in the laundry bag.
19. Wash your hands.
20. Report to the nurse that you have given the patient a heat lamp treatment and your observations of the patient's skin condition.

General Rules for Cold Applications

- Always use a bath thermometer to check the temperature of cold moist applications.
- Always use the temperature instructed for the patient. Pay special attention with elderly patients, infants, and others more susceptible to cold injury.
- Always carefully time the cold application and never exceed the instructed length.
- Monitor the patient carefully and immediately report any signs of problems or patient complaints of pain or numbness.
- Explain to the patient the purpose of the cold application and the risks; do not let the patient change the temperature level or length of the application.
- Use ice cubes rather than crushed ice, which may melt too fast.
- Do not cover a cold application once applied, as a cover may trap heat beneath it.

PROCEDURE: GIVING A COOLING SPONGE BATH

1. Wash your hands.
2. Check the patient's identification bracelet and speak the patient's name.
3. Explain to the patient that you are going to give a cooling sponge bath.
4. Follow facility policy for asking visitors to leave the room.

5. Collect the following equipment: bath basin, an equal mixture of cool water and 70% rubbing alcohol, bath thermometer, six ice bags with flannel covers, bath blanket, bath towels, a hand towel, two washcloths, waterproof bed protector, thermometer, sphygmomanometer, and stethoscope. Follow facility policy whether to use alcohol or water in the sponge bath.
6. Close the privacy curtain and the room door.
7. Take the patient's temperature, pulse, respiration, and blood pressure and record the results and time.
8. Raise the bed to a high level to ease your body movements.
9. Lower the near side rail.
10. Spread the bath blanket over the patient. Reaching under the bath blanket, fold the top linens to the foot of the bed.
11. Reaching under the bath blanket, remove the patient's gown.
12. Turn the patient to the side and slip the waterproof bed protector under the body.
13. Raise the side rail.
14. Slip the ice bags in the flannel covers and fill them with ice.
15. Slip the hot water bag in a flannel cover and follow instructions for filling it.
16. Lower the near side rail, and help the patient move to the side of the bed.
17. Place an ice bag on each side of the patient's neck, on the forehead, in each armpit, and on the groin. Place the hot water bottle at the patient's feet.

18. Prepare one hand towel as a cold compress and place it under the patient's knees.
19. Raise the side rail.
20. Fill the wash basin two-thirds with the cool (68 to 86 degrees F or 20 to 30 degrees C) water and alcohol mixture, testing the temperature with the bath thermometer.
21. Put both washcloths into the wash basin.
22. Lower the side rail.
23. Place a bath towel under the patient's far arm.
24. Make a mitt with a washcloth and sponge the patient's arm with long, gentle strokes. Alternate the washcloths. Pat dry.
25. Place a bath towel under the patient's near arm and sponge it in the same way.
26. Place a bath towel lengthwise on the chest and groin. Reaching under the towel, fold the bath blanket down to the edge of the towel without exposing the patient.
27. Sponge the chest, abdomen, and groin with the washcloths in the same way. Pat dry.
28. Measure the patient's vital signs, and record the results and time.
29. If the patient shivers, shows signs of cyanosis (turning blue), or complains of feeling cold, stop the sponging and notify the nurse immediately.
30. Place a bath towel under the far leg.
31. Sponge the leg with the wet washcloths with long, gentle strokes. Pat dry and cover with the bath blanket.
32. Place a bath towel under the patient's near leg and sponge it in the same way.
33. Help the patient turn onto the side facing away from you, taking care not to expose the body.

34. Place a bath towel on the bed along the patient's back.
35. Sponge the back and buttocks with long, gentle strokes. Pat dry.
36. When the treatment is done, remove the ice bags, hot water bottle, towels, and waterproof bed protector.
37. Help the patient resume a comfortable position. Measure the patient's vital signs, and record the results and time.
38. Put a clean gown on the patient and remove the bath blanket. Make the bed, replacing any wet linens.
39. Lower the bed to a safe and comfortable position.
40. Make sure the side rails are raised and the patient can reach the signal light.
41. Open the privacy curtain and room door.
42. Clean and return equipment to its proper location, and discard and trash. Place soiled linens in the laundry bag.
43. Measure the patient's vital signs 10 and 30 minutes after the treatment. Record the results and the time.
44. Wash your hands.
45. Report to the nurse that you have given the patient a cooling sponge bath, the vital signs taken before, during, and after the treatment, and how well the patient tolerated the procedure.

PROCEDURE: APPLYING A COLD COMPRESS

1. Wash your hands.
2. Check the patient's identification bracelet and speak the patient's name.
3. Explain to the patient that you are going to apply a cold compress.
4. Follow facility policy for asking visitors to leave the room.
5. Collect wash basin with ice, pitcher filled with cold water, waterproof bed protector, washcloths or gauze pads, bath blanket, and bath towel.
6. Close the privacy curtain.
7. Raise the bed to a high level to ease your body movements.
8. Place the pitcher of water in the ice basin.
9. Lower the side rail.
10. Place the waterproof bed protector under the body area to be treated. Make sure the patient is comfortable.
11. Place the washcloths or gauze pads in the pitcher, and wring them out thoroughly as you use them.
12. Apply the compress to the proper area, noting the time.
13. To ensure that the patient does not become chilled, spread a bath blanket over the body, leaving the treated area uncovered.
14. Check the treated area every 5 minutes for blisters, pale or white skin, cyanosis (blue skin), or shivering. If these problems occur, or if the patient complains of pain or numbness, stop the treatment and report the problem to the nurse immediately.

15. Change the compress if it becomes warm.
16. After 20 minutes, remove the compress and dry the area with the bath towel. Remove the bath blanket.
17. Lower the bed to a safe and comfortable position.
18. Make sure the side rails are raised and the patient can reach the signal light.
19. Open the privacy curtain.
20. Return equipment to its proper location, and discard soiled linens in the laundry bag.
21. Wash your hands.
22. Report to the nurse that you have applied a cold compress and your observations of the patient's skin condition.

PROCEDURE: GIVING A COLD SOAK

1. Wash your hands.
2. Check the patient's identification bracelet and speak the patient's name.
3. Explain to the patient that you are going to give a cold soak.
4. Follow facility policy for asking visitors to leave the room.
5. Collect the following equipment: wash basin or foot or arm basin, pitcher of cold water, bath blanket, towels, and waterproof bed protector.
6. Close the privacy curtain.
7. Raise the bed to a high level to ease your body movements. Help the patient assume a comfortable position.
8. Place a waterproof bed protector under the body area to be treated.

9. Fill the basin halfway with cold water from the pitcher.
10. Expose the body area to be treated.
11. Slowly place the hand, foot, or arm into the basin, noting the time the treatment begins.
12. Cover the patient with the bath blanket.
13. Every 5 minutes, check the water temperature and change it if it becomes warm.
14. Every 5 minutes, check the treated area for whiteness or discoloration. If this occurs, or if the patient complains of weakness or feeling cold, stop the treatment and cover the treated area with a towel. Report the problem to the nurse immediately.
15. When the treatment is complete, remove the extremity from the water and dry it with a towel. Remove the bath blanket.
16. Lower the bed to a safe and comfortable position.
17. Make sure the side rails are raised and the patient can reach the signal light.
18. Open the privacy curtain.
19. Return equipment to its proper location, and put soiled linens in the laundry bag.
20. Wash your hands.
21. Report to the nurse that you have given the patient a cold soak and your observations of the patient's skin condition.

PROCEDURE: APPLYING AN ICE BAG

1. Wash your hands.
2. Check the patient's identification bracelet and speak the patient's name.

3. Explain to the patient that you are going to apply an ice bag.
4. Follow facility policy for asking visitors to leave the room.
5. Collect the following equipment: ice bag, ice cap, or ice collar, flannel cover, ice cubes, bath blanket, and paper towels.
6. Close the privacy curtain.
7. Raise the bed to a high level to ease your body movements. Help the patient assume a comfortable position.
8. To check the ice bag for leaks, pour water into it, close it, and turn it upside down.
9. Fill the bag halfway with ice cubes.
10. To force air from the bag, squeeze the sides with your hands. Fasten the stopper tightly.
11. Dry the outside of the bag with paper towels.
12. Place the flannel cover on the bag.
13. Place the bag on the prescribed body part, noting the time the treatment begins.
14. Cover the patient with the bath blanket.
15. Make sure the patient can reach the signal light.
16. Check the skin under the bag every 10 minutes for blisters, pale, white or grey skin, cyanosis (blue skin), or shivering. If these problems occur, or if the patient complains of numbness, pain, or burning, remove the bag. Report the problem to the nurse immediately.
17. Remove the bag after the prescribed time.
18. Lower the bed to a safe and comfortable position.
19. Make sure the side rails are raised and the patient can reach the signal light.
20. Open the privacy curtain.

21. Return equipment to its proper location, and discard any trash. Place soiled linens in the laundry bag.
22. Wash your hands.
23. Report to the nurse that you have applied an ice bag to the patient and your observations of the patient's skin condition.

PROCEDURE: APPLYING A DISPOSABLE COLD PACK

1. Wash your hands.
2. Check the patient's identification bracelet and speak the patient's name.
3. Explain to the patient that you are going to apply a cold pack.
4. Follow facility policy for asking visitors to leave the room.
5. Collect the following equipment: a commercial cold pack, flannel cover, tape or rolled gauze, and bath blanket.
6. Close the privacy curtain.
7. Raise the bed to ease your body movements. Help the patient assume a comfortable position.
8. To activate the cold pack, strike or squeeze it as the instructions indicate.
9. Place the flannel cover on the pack.
10. Place the pack on the prescribed body part, noting the time the treatment begins.
11. Fasten the pack with the tape or rolled gauze.
12. Cover the patient with the bath blanket.
13. Make sure the patient can reach the signal light.

14. Every 10 minutes, check the skin under the pack for blisters, white, pale, or grey skin, cyanosis (blue skin), or shivering. If these problems occur, or if the patient complains of numbness, pain, or burning, stop the treatment. Report the problem to the nurse immediately.
15. Remove the bag after the prescribed length of treatment. Remove the bath blanket.
16. Lower the bed to a safe and comfortable position.
17. Make sure the side rails are raised and the patient can reach the signal light.
18. Open the privacy curtain.
19. Discard disposable equipment and trash, and put soiled linens in the laundry bag.
20. Wash your hands.
21. Report to the nurse that you have applied a cold pack to the patient and your observations of the patient's skin condition.

Chapter 13
Exercise and Activity

This chapter includes information on the following:
General rules for exercising patients
Procedure: Helping patient with range-of-motion
exercises
Procedure: Helping the patient walk

General Rules for Exercising Patients

- When you assist the patient with range-of-motion exercises or walking, be sure to follow orders in the amount and type of exercise.
- Be alert to the patient's response to exercise and stop immediately if the patient complains of pain or fatigue.
- When assisting the patient, pay attention to your own body mechanics and alignment.
- Move joints smoothly and gently and do not force a joint it you feel resistance in the range of motion.
- Never force any movement if it is painful for the patient.
- Always explain the exercise to the patient and encourage the patient to move the joints as much as possible without your assistance.
- Report to the nurse any patient complaints of pain or serious discomfort experienced during exercise.
- When walking the patient, be sure the area is free of any clutter on the floor. Make sure there is a chair at a resting point. Use a transfer belt for a patient at risk of falling.

- If the patient is using a walker or cane, be sure it is in good condition and has a nonskid rubber tip.

PROCEDURE: HELPING PATIENT WITH RANGE-OF-MOTION EXERCISES

1. Wash your hands.
2. Check the patient's identification bracelet and speak the patient's name.
3. Explain that you are going help the patient perform range-of-motion exercises. If this is the first time, explain the value of these exercises for the patient.
4. Follow facility policy for asking visitors to leave the room.
5. Obtain a bath blanket.
6. Close the privacy curtain.
7. Raise the bed to a high level to ease your body movements. Lower the side rail.
8. Help the patient into the supine position, on the back with arms at sides and legs extended.
9. Cover the patient with the bath blanket and fold the top bed linens to the foot of the bed.
10. Follow a systematic head-to-toe order for the exercises. Repeat each of the following exercises 3 to 5 times or as ordered.
11. Exercise the neck:
    a. With hands at sides over ears, support the head.
    b. Flex the neck by moving the head forward until the chin touches the chest, then move it back to the pillow.

    c. Rotate the neck by turning the head to the left and right.

    d. Laterally flex the neck by tipping the top of the head to the left and right.

    e. Repeat the sequence.

12. Exercise each shoulder:

    a. Support the arm with one hand at the wrist and the other at the elbow.

    b. Flex the shoulder by lifting the arm toward the ceiling and over the head; slowly return the arm toward the center of the body.

    c. Hyperextend the shoulder if the patient is sitting up: move the arm behind the body and then back.

    d. Abduct the shoulder by moving the arm straight out from the side; return it slowly to the side.

    e. Rotate the shoulder by moving the arm out to the side at shoulder level; bring the hand forward to touch the bed palm down, then move backward to shoulder level.

    f. Repeat the sequence.

13. Exercise each elbow:

    a. Support the elbow by holding the wrist with one hand and the elbow with the other.

    b. Flex the elbow by bending the arm to bring the hand to the shoulder; slowly straighten the arm.

    c. Pronate the elbow by holding the hand in handshake position and turn the hand palm down and then up.

    d. Repeat the sequence.

14. Exercise each wrist:

    a. Support the forearm with one hand and the hand with the other.

    b. Flex the wrist by bending the hand forward; then slowly hyperextend it by moving it backward.

    c. Move the hand from side to side at the wrist.

    d. Repeat the sequence.

15. Exercise the fingers of each hand:

    a. Support the hand at the wrist.

    b. Flex the fingers by bringing them in to make a fist; then extend the fingers straight out.

    c. Abduct the fingers and thumb by spreading them out sideways from each other; adduct them by moving them back together.

    d. Flex the thumb by bending it to the base of the little finger; then extend it back out to the side.

    e. Oppose the thumb by moving it to touch the tip of each of the fingers.

    f. Repeat the sequence.

16. Exercise each hip:

    a. Support the leg by holding under the knee with one hand and under the ankle with the other.

    b. Flex the hip by raising the leg up from the bed; lower it slowly back.

    c. Abduct the hip by moving the leg out to the side; bring it slowly back.

    d. Rotate the hip internally by turning the foot so that the toes are toward the other leg; rotate the leg externally by turning the foot away from the other foot.

    e. Repeat the sequence.

17. Exercise each knee:
    a. Support the leg with one hand under the knee and the other under the ankle.
    b. Flex the knee by raising the leg up from the bed and bending the knee; extend it slowly back out straight.
    c. Repeat the sequence.
18. Exercise each ankle:
    a. Support the ankle with the foot in one hand and the ankle in the other.
    b. Invert the foot by turning it sideways so that the bottom of the foot tilts toward the other foot; evert the foot by turning it sideways so that the bottom tilts away from the other foot.
    c. Dorsiflex the ankle by bending the foot with toes back toward the leg; plantarflex the ankle by pointing the toes downward.
    d. Repeat the sequence.
19. Exercise the toes of each foot:
    a. Support the foot in both hands.
    b. Flex the toes by curling them in; extend them out straight.
    c. Abduct the toes by spreading them out away from each other; adduct them by bringing them back together.
    d. Repeat the sequence.
20. Return the patient to a comfortable position.
21. Fold the top bed linens back up and remove the bath blanket.
22. Raise the side rail. Lower the bed to its lowest horizontal position.
23 Make sure the patient is comfortable and can reach the signal light.
24. Open the privacy curtain.

25. Wash your hands.
26. Report to the nurse that you have helped the patient with range-of-motion exercises, how the activity was tolerated, and any unusual observations.

PROCEDURE: HELPING THE PATIENT WALK

1. Wash your hands.
2. Check the patient's identification bracelet and speak the patient's name.
3. Explain to the patient that you are going to help the patient walk and that the transfer belt (also called a gait belt) is a safety precaution.
4. Obtain a transfer belt.
5. Close the privacy curtain.
6. Lower the bed to its lowest horizontal position. Lower the side rail. Lock the bed wheels.
7. Help the patient to sit on the side of the bed (see Chapter 6 procedure) and regain a sense of balance.
8. Help the patient put on slippers or shoes and socks and robe.
9. Put the transfer belt on the patient (see Chapter 6 procedure).
10. Make sure no furniture or equipment is in the way before you help the patient stand.
11. Help the patient stand up: the patient pushes down with hands on the mattress as you assist by lifting with one hand on each side of the transfer belt.
12. Let the patient regain a sense of balance; stand at one side, with one hand on the belt at that side and the other hand on the belt at the patient's back.

13. Ask the patient to stand with head and back straight in good body alignment, facing straight ahead.
14. With both hands on the belt, standing on the patient's weak side, help the patient walk as normal as possible. Move your feet in the same pattern as the patients': left foot together, right foot together.
15. Ask the patient if able to fully raise each foot and bring it to the floor heel first rather than sliding or shuffling feet.
16. Walk the patient the ordered distance, at the patient's pace--do not hurry the patient.
17. Return the patient to the chair or bed and to sit down, keeping both hands on the transfer belt.
18. Remove the transfer belt, robe, and slippers. Help the patient lie down in bed (see Chapter 6).
19. Adjust the bed linens. Raise the side rail.
20. Make sure the patient is comfortable and can reach the signal light.
21. Open the privacy curtain.
22. Wash your hands.
23. Report to the nurse that you have helped the patient walk, how the patient tolerated the activity, and any unusual observations.

Chapter 14
Rehabilitation

This chapter includes information on the following:
Principles of rehabilitation
General rules for helping rehabilitate patients

Principles of Rehabilitation

- Because the goal of rehabilitation is to restore the patient to functioning as independently as possible, always involve the patient as much as possible in care activities.
- Give emotional support and encouragement for even small amounts of progress; help the patient focus on abilities rather than disabilities. Always look at the positive side.
- Help the patient with range-of-motion exercises as ordered (see Chapter 13 procedure) and encourage the patient to take an active role in these exercises.
- Because an immobile or inactive patient is more susceptible to bedsores, observe carefully for the first signs of bedsores and report any signs to the nurse; use preventive methods (see Chapter 7).
- Help the patient maintain good body alignment in bed and when sitting.
- Try to motivate the patient to do as much self-care as possible, such as personal hygiene.
- Try to involve the patient in social and recreational activities appropriate for the patient's condition.

▸ Take an active interest in all aspects of the patient's rehabilitation program and assist as needed with other therapies such as physical therapy; be able to help with any special equipment the patient is using.

▸ Report to the nurse any change in the patient's behavior, condition, or emotional attitude.

General Rules for Helping Rehabilitate Patients

■ When feeding a disabled patient:
- Allow the patient to eat and drink as independently as possible; help only as needed.
- Use special utensils when appropriate that are easier to handle; use cups with handles or straws.
- Serve food that can be easily chewed and swallowed.
- Make the meal experience as pleasant as possible, with attractively arranged meal tray and no clutter or distractions present in the room.
- Allow family and other visitors to join the patient when eating.
- When appropriate you may have pleasant conversation with the patient while eating.
- With a patient who has a sensory problem or is disoriented, observe that the patient is chewing and swallowing well; be alert for possible choking.

■ When helping a disabled patient to bathe:
- Allow and encourage the patient to be as independent as possible in washing.
- Let the patient wash areas the patient can reach; you wash the areas beyond reach.

- If you are unfamiliar with a particular disability, talk with the nurse or physical therapist before beginning to bathe or otherwise assist the patient physically.
- Always make sure the environment is safe for the patient. Keep equipment and supplies for personal hygiene where the patient can reach it. Put the soap bar on a sponge or wash cloth so that it doesn't slide from the patient's grasp.
- Never leave the patient alone in the middle of a procedure.
- Never rush the patient or give the patient any sense of being in a hurry to complete bathing or any procedure.
- If so instructed, wash the disabled arm or leg first.
- When helping a disabled patient to dress:
  - For good emotional health encourage the patient to dress in street clothes rather than stay in pajamas or gown all the time.
  - Allow and encourage the patient to be as independent as possible in undressing and dressing. Let the patient choose the clothes to wear. Assist with dressing and undressing only as needed.
  - Dress the weakest or disabled arm or leg first.
  - Never leave the patient alone in the middle of getting dressed or undressed.
  - Never rush the patient or give the patient any sense of being in a hurry when dressing or undressing.

Encourage the patient to groom himself or herself with home habits; let the female patient use makeup as preferred.

Chapter 15
Special Procedures

This chapter includes information on the following:
General rules for patients on oxygen therapy
General rules for care of an IV
Procedure: Use of elastic stockings
Procedure: Use of elastic bandages
Procedure: Applying an arm sling bandage
Procedure: Preparing the patient for physical
examination
Procedure: Collecting a sputum specimen

General Rules for Patients on Oxygen Therapy

■ Carefully follow safety precautions to prevent
  fires whenever oxygen is being used:
  - Be sure "no smoking" signs are posted and
    all visitors are aware of this.
  - Before bringing any electrical equipment into
    the room, test it to be sure it is functioning
    properly and does not cause sparks.
  - Do not unplug electrical equipment while
    turned on, as a spark may result at the plug.
  - Avoid use of wool and synthetic fabrics that
    may make sparks of static electricity.
  - Avoid use of flammable materials such as
    petroleum jelly, rubbing alcohol, and nail
    polish remover.
■ Never interrupt the flow of oxygen by removing
  the oxygen delivery device or turning off the
  tank or wall outlet.
■ Periodically check the oxygen flow:
  - Look for any twists or kinks in the tubing.

- Make sure the patient is not lying on the tubing.
- Check the gauge on the oxygen tank and report to the nurse if it is low.
- Check the flowmeter on the oxygen tank and report to the nurse if it is not delivering oxygen at the correct rate.

■ Be sure oxygen tanks are secured by straps or other means to prevent them from falling.

■ If a humidifying jar is used in the oxygen line, check the water level to ensure it bubbles as the oxygen passes through.

■ Observe the patient for any signs of difficulty breathing and report any unusual signs to the nurse immediately.

■ Check the elastic band on a face mask or cannula to be sure it is not too tight and causing a pressure area; look for any areas of irritation around the mask.

■ Since oxygen dries mouth tissues, provide fluids and oral hygiene often.

General Rules for Care of an IV

■ Check the IV system frequently to make sure the fluid is flowing properly out of the bag or bottle, through the drip chamber, and through the tubing. Do not try to adjust the flow but report any problem to the nurse.

■ Look for any twists or kinks in the tubing.

■ Make sure the patient is not lying on the tubing.

■ Check the area around the needle and report to the nurse any redness, bleeding, swelling, or pain.

PROCEDURE: USE OF ELASTIC STOCKINGS

1. Wash your hands.
2. Check the patient's identification bracelet and speak the patient's name.
3. Explain to the patient that you are going to apply elastic stockings. If this is the first time for the patient, explain the stockings are to promote good blood flow.
4. Follow facility policy for asking visitors to leave the room.
5. Obtain elastic stockings in the size the nurse orders.
6. Close the privacy curtain.
7. Raise the bed to a high level to ease your body movements. Lower the side rail.
8. Position the patient lying flat on the back (supine position).
9. Fold the top bed linens toward the patient's waist to expose the legs.
10. Gather up the top of the stocking and turn the stocking inside out down to the heel area to make it easier to insert the foot.
11. Holding the patient's foot at the heel, slide the foot of the stocking over the patient's foot.
12. Straighten any wrinkles in the foot and position it snugly; then pull the stocking up over the leg.
13. Straighten the stocking and remove any wrinkles.
14. Repeat the process for the other leg.
15. Fold the top bed linens back down to the foot of the bed.
16. Raise the side rail. Lower the bed to its lowest horizontal position.

17. Make sure the patient is comfortable and can reach the signal light.
18. Open the privacy curtain.
19. Wash your hands.
20. Report to the nurse that you have applied the stockings and any unusual observations.
21. Because elastic stockings are usually removed in no more than 8 hours, confirm with the nurse whether you are to remove them later.

PROCEDURE: USE OF ELASTIC BANDAGES

1. Wash your hands.
2. Check the patient's identification bracelet and speak the patient's name.
3. Explain to the patient that you are going to apply an elastic bandage. If this is the first time for the patient, explain the bandage is to promote good blood flow and provide support.
4. Follow facility policy for asking visitors to leave the room.
5. Obtain the elastic bandage in the length and width the nurse orders.
6. Close the privacy curtain.
7. Raise the bed to a high level to ease your body movements. Lower the side rail.
8. Position the patient lying flat on the back (supine position) or in a comfortable position that allows you to work with the arm or leg to be wrapped.
9. Expose the leg or arm to be wrapped and make sure it is clean and dry.
10. Extend the arm or leg straight out and support the wrist or heel.

11. Holding the rolled bandage so that the free end comes off the bottom, make two turns around the smallest part of the section to be bandaged (wrist, ankle, knee) to anchor the bandage.
12. Roll the bandage upward around the arm or leg, smoothly and firmly but not tightly, with each turn overlapping about half of the previous turn.
13. Clip or pin the end of the bandage in place, or if continuing with a second bandage overlap the second to keep the end of the first in place.
14. Raise the side rail. Lower the bed to its lowest horizontal position.
15. Make sure the patient is comfortable and can reach the signal light.
16. Open the privacy curtain.
17. Wash your hands.
18. Report to the nurse that you have applied the stockings and any unusual observations.
19. Check frequently to see if the patient's fingers or toes are cold or look bluish; ask whether the patient feels any pain or numbness. With any of these, remove the bandage and report the problem to the nurse.
20. Since the bandage is usually removed in no more than 8 hours, confirm with the nurse whether you are to remove the bandage later.

PROCEDURE: APPLYING AN ARM SLING BANDAGE

1. Wash your hands.
2. Check the patient's identification bracelet and speak the patient's name.
3. Explain to the patient what you are going to do.
4. Follow facility policy for asking visitors to leave the room.
5. Obtain a bandage of triangular material or square shape folded into a triangle and a pin.
6. Close the privacy curtain.
7. Raise the bed to a high level to ease your body movements. Lower the side rail.
8. Help the patient sit on the side of the bed (see Chapter 6 procedure).
9. Position the bandage with one end of the triangle over the shoulder on the noninjured side and the side point of the triangle beneath the elbow.
10. Gently position the injured arm across the chest and bring the lower corner up and over the shoulder on the injured side.
11. Adjust the length of the sling so that the hand is slightly higher than the elbow and the hand and wrist are supported.
12. Tie the two ends of the sling at the side of the neck with a square knot.
13. Check the patient's hand and arm often to make sure there are no pain or signs of poor circulation (cold skin, bluish color in the hand).
14. Help the patient lie back in bed.
15. Raise the side rail. Lower the bed to its lowest horizontal position.

16. Make sure the patient is comfortable and can reach the signal light.
17. Open the privacy curtain.
18. Wash your hands.
19. Report to the nurse that you have made a sling bandage for the patient and any unusual observations.

PROCEDURE: PREPARING THE PATIENT FOR PHYSICAL EXAMINATION

1. Wash your hands.
2. Check the patient's identification bracelet and speak the patient's name.
3. Explain that you are preparing the patient for a physical examination by the nurse, doctor, or other examiner.
4. Follow facility policy for asking visitors to leave the room.
5. Prepare the following equipment on a tray by the bed: gown, disposable gloves, towel, bath blanket, bed protector, drape, emesis basin, tissues, paper towels, cotton balls, cotton-tip swabs, alcohol wipes, thermometer, blood pressure cuff, stethoscope, throat mirror, flashlight, tongue depressors, nasal speculum, reflex hammer, tuning fork, specimen jars with labels, microscope slides, paper and pen, disposable bag, otoscope, and ophthalmoscope.
6. Close the privacy curtain.
7. Ask the patient to put on the gown. Help the patient as needed (see Chapter 7 procedure).

8.   Ask the patient to urinate and/or defecate if able. Offer a bedpan or urinal if the patient cannot use the bathroom (see Chapter 11 procedures).
9.   Help the patient to lie back in bed.
10. Raise the bed to the highest level. Lower the side rail.
11. Put the bed protector under the patient's hips and buttocks, and drape the patient.
12. Use the signal light to call the nurse or examiner. Raise the side rail if you leave the room to get the examiner.
13. Assist as requested during the examination.
14. After the examination, put away equipment and dispose of used supplies. Help the patient dress and become comfortable in bed.
15. Raise the side rail. Lower the bed to its lowest horizontal position.
16. Make sure the patient is comfortable and can reach the signal light.
17. Open the privacy curtain.
18. Wash your hands.
19. Report to the nurse that the patient is back in bed after the examination and any unusual observations.

PROCEDURE: COLLECTING A SPUTUM SPECIMEN

1.   Wash your hands.
2.   Check the patient's identification bracelet and speak the patient's name.
3.   Explain that you need to collect a sputum specimen from the patient and what the patient needs to do.

4. Follow facility policy for asking visitors to leave the room.
5. Collect the following equipment: specimen container with lid and label, pen, tissues, and disposable gloves.
6. Close the privacy curtain.
7. Prepare the specimen label with information from the patient's identification bracelet.
8. Ask the patient to rinse the mouth with water; oral hygiene is optional.
9. Help the patient sit up in bed if able (see Chapter 6 procedure).
10. Put on the disposable gloves. Give the sputum specimen container to the patient and explain what to do: cover the nose with tissues, take two or three deep breaths, and cough deep to bring up sputum: cough it directly into the container.
11. Repeat as necessary to collect 1 to 2 tablespoons of sputum.
12. Put the lid on the specimen container immediately, being careful not to touch inside the container or lid.
13. Take or send the specimen immediately to the laboratory.
14. Remove the disposable gloves. Help the patient lie back down (see Chapter 6 procedure).
15. Make sure the bed is lowered to its lowest horizontal position and the side rails are up.
16. Make sure the patient is comfortable and can reach the signal light.
17. Open the privacy curtain.
18. Wash your hands.

19. Report to the nurse that you have collected the sputum specimen, the appearance and consistency of the sputum, how easily the patient coughed up the sputum, and any unusual observations.

Chapter 16
The Orthopedic Patient

This chapter includes information on the following:
Principles of care
General rules for skin care
General rules for traction care
General rules for cast care
Procedure: Using a turning frame

Principles of Care

► Never use special orthopedic equipment until you become fully familiar with its proper use.
► Nursing care must be adapted to orthopedic patients to perform all procedures without disturbing orthopedic equipment such as casts, splints, prosthetic devices, braces, crutches, and so on.
► Because the orthopedic patient may be immobile for long periods, position changes and skin care are very important.
► Because orthopedic injuries often heal very slowly, the patient may be depressed or frustrated and thus needs special understanding and encouragement.

General Rules for Skin Care

■ Depending on the doctor's orders, change the patient's position every two hours or as instructed.
■ Provide backrubs frequently (as ordered) (see Chapter 7 procedure).

- Keep the bed dry and clean and the linen free of wrinkles.
- Provide good cleaning of the skin and cast at the edge of the cast, to prevent itching.
- Follow the principles for preventing bedsores (see Chapter 7).
- Encourage patients in casts to use the trapeze bar for movement and to help you when changing their position.

General Rules for Traction Care

- If the traction patient complains of pain or discomfort, or of tingling or numbness in the arm or leg in a cast, report it to the nurse immediately.
- Do not change the patient's body position without having been ordered to do so.
- Provide frequent skin care for a patient in traction (see above). Observe the skin color near the cast or splint and immediately report any discoloration.
- If the traction is to be continuous (not intermittent), never interrupt the system of weights, ropes, and pulleys.
- Observe the positioning of the patient and traction system and report any of the following problems:
  - The patient having slid down in bed.
  - The weights on the floor.
  - The splinted leg or arm out of position.
  - The rope off the pulley.
  - Weights that are not evenly balanced.
- Follow the general rules for cast care (see following section).

General Rules for Cast Care

- When the cast is drying, do not cover it with a blanket or other covering; do not move the patient during the drying. If it is necessary to touch the cast while it is drying, do so only with the palm of your hand.
- Keep the bed side rails up for a patient with a cast.
- Be careful not to soil the cast when providing hygiene and other care and when helping the patient with a bedpan or urinal. Protect the cast from becoming wet.
- Provide frequent skin care for a patient in a cast (see above). Observe the skin near a cast or splint and immediately report any discoloration, swelling, or cool or hot skin areas.
- If the patient complains of pain or discomfort, or of tingling or numbness in the arm or leg in a cast, report it to the nurse immediately.
- Report immediately any unusual smells coming from the cast, which may indicate an infection under the cast.
- Unless ordered otherwise, elevate the arm or leg in a cast by supporting it on pillows to reduce swelling.
- Get assistance when repositioning a patient in a cast, which may affect the patient's balance and require additional strength to move the patient.
- Although the patient may complain of itching beneath the cast, do not let the patient use any object to try to scratch under the cast, because skin injuries and infection may result.

PROCEDURE: USING A TURNING FRAME

1. Wash your hands.
2. Check the patient's identification bracelet and speak the patient's name.
3. Explain that you are going to turn the patient on the turning frame.
4. Follow facility policy for asking visitors to leave the room.
5. Have ready the top and bottom parts of the frame, a bath blanket, a sheepskin or other padded covering, and two others to assist you.
6. Close the privacy curtain.
7. Cover the patient with the bath blanket and remove the gown.
8. Remove the foot support and arm boards; put the patient's arms along the sides.
9. Cover the patient with the sheepskin or other covering.
10. Position the top section of the frame over the sheepskin or other covering.
11. Position the head and face support section for a proper fit, and lock the top frame in place. Position security straps at the knees, hips, and shoulders.
12. With two others assisting you, standing at one side facing the frame, turn the patient by rotating the frames so that the bottom frame is now on top.
13. Be sure the frame is securely in place and remove the security straps and the frame now on top.
14. Position the arm boards and foot support.

15. Make sure the patient is comfortable on top of the sheepskin or other material. Cover the patient with a sheet.
16. Make sure the patient can reach the signal light.
17. Open the privacy curtain.
18. Wash your hands.
19. Report to the nurse that you have turned the patient and any unusual observations.

Chapter 17
The Surgical Patient

This chapter includes information on the following:
Principles of preoperative care
Procedure: Shaving the skin for surgery
Principles of postoperative care
Procedure: Assisting the patient with coughing
and deep breathing
Procedure: Assisting the patient with leg
exercises

Principles of Preoperative Care

- ▶ Be supportive and encouraging and listen to the patient's concerns, but let the nurse or doctor answer any questions about the surgery.
- ▶ All health professionals caring for the patient are involved in patient education before the surgery to prepare the patient for what to expect.
- ▶ In the period preceding the surgery observe the patient carefully and report signs of infection, sneezing or coughing, complaints of pain, or changed vital signs.
- ▶ Follow all instructions carefully and exactly, such as to keep the patient NPO (nothing by mouth--no food or drink) after a specified time, removal of jewelry, hygiene procedures, and so on.
- ▶ Most facilities use a preoperative checklist for nursing care, and your responsibilities on this list will be outlined for you.

PROCEDURE: SHAVING THE SKIN FOR SURGERY

1. Wash your hands.
2. Check the patient's identification bracelet and speak the patient's name.
3. Explain to the patient that you are going to shave the skin around the surgical site to prepare for the operation.
4. Follow facility policy for asking visitors to leave the room.
5. Collect the following equipment: disposable skin prep kit (with razor, razor blades, soap sponge, plastic basin, and paper towels), bath blanket, bath thermometer, bed protector, and bath towel.
6. Close the privacy curtain.
7. Raise the bed to a high level to ease your body movements. Lower the side rail.
8. Put the bath blanket over the patient and fold the top bed linens down to the foot of the bed without exposing the patient.
9. Put the bed protector under the area to be shaved.
10. Position the bedside lamp to light the area directly.
11. Open the disposable skin prep kit. Use the plastic container as a basin and fill it with warm water (115 degrees F, or 46 degrees C), using the bath thermometer.
12. Pull back the bath blanket to expose the area to be shaved.
13. Using the soap sponge and warm water, soap the area to be shaved and make a lather.

14. Holding the razor in one hand, use the fingers of the other hand to keep the skin taut. Shave in short firm strokes in the direction of hair growth. Rinse the razor often in the basin. Add more soap and lather as needed while shaving to keep the skin always wet.
15. Check to make sure the whole area is shaved thoroughly.
16. Put fresh warm water in the basin and rinse the skin
17. Pat the skin dry with the towel.
18. Remove the bed protector and cover the patient with the bath blanket.
19. Fold the bed top linens back up and remove the bath blanket.
20. Raise the side rail. Lower the bed to its lowest horizontal position.
21. Make sure the patient is comfortable and can reach the signal light.
22. Open the privacy curtain.
23. Dispose of the used equipment and dirty laundry.
24. Wash your hands.
25. Report to the nurse that you have shaved the patient for surgery and any unusual observations. Report any nicks or scratches in the patient's skin.

Principles of Postoperative Care

► Prepare the room before the patient returns from surgery:
  • Make a surgical bed (see Chapter 5 procedure). Have the bed ready with rails down and in the highest horizontal position.

- • Collect equipment for measuring vital signs, IV hanger pole, and other standard room equipment (see Chapter 4).
- • Have furniture out of the way and the bedside area clear for the stretcher's arrival.
► Assist the nurse when the patient arrives in the room:
  - • Help transfer the patient from the stretcher to the bed and position the patient in bed.
  - • Be sure the side rails are raised and the signal light is within reach.
  - • Cover the patient with a blanket as instructed.
  - • Assist in taking vital signs as instructed (see Chapter 9 procedures).
► Check on the patient frequently in the postoperative period. Report to the nurse:
  - • Any change in vital signs.
  - • Patient complaints of pain, nausea, or thirst.
  - • Bleeding or increased drainage in dressings.
  - • Changes in skin color or temperature.
  - • Vomiting or choking.
  - • Patient restlessness or confusion.
► Position the patient only as instructed:
  - • The position should not impede easy breathing or disturb the surgical site.
  - • Usually the patient is repositioned every 2 hours, taking care to minimize pain and discomfort.
► Assist the patient with coughing, deep breathing, and leg exercises as instructed (see following procedures).
► Provide emotional support and encouragement throughout the postoperative period.

PROCEDURE: ASSISTING THE PATIENT WITH COUGHING AND DEEP BREATHING

1. Wash your hands.
2. Check the patient's identification bracelet and speak the patient's name.
3. Explain that you are going to help the patient cough and breathe deeply to help prevent respiratory complications after surgery.
4. Follow facility policy for asking visitors to leave the room.
5. Have ready a pillow, disposable bag, and tissues.
6. Close the privacy curtain.
7. Raise the bed to a high level to ease your body movements. Lower the side rail.
8. Let the patient use the bedpan or urinal if needed (see Chapter 11 procedures).
9. Help the patient to sit on the side of the bed if allowed or to sit up in bed (see Chapter 6 procedures).
10. If the patient's incision is over the abdomen, position the pillow over this site; otherwise position the pillow over the lower ribs. Ask the patient to hold the pillow firmly in place.
11. Ask the patient to take a deep breath in through the nose and to hold it in for a second or two before exhaling through the mouth slowly and deeply.
12. Ask the patient to breathe in and out as deeply as possible for 5 to 10 times, as instructed. Encourage the patient to breathe deeply even if feeling mild discomfort.

13. Ask the patient to hold the pillow over the incision site and to cough with mouth open into the tissues. Encourage the patient to cough strongly enough to remove secretions.
14. Help the patient to return to the original position, and reposition the pillow.
15. Raise the side rail. Lower the bed to its lowest horizontal position.
16. Make sure the patient is comfortable and can reach the signal light.
17. Dispose of the used tissues in the disposable bag.
18. Open the privacy curtain.
19. Wash your hands.
20. Report to the nurse that you have helped the patient cough and breathe deeply, the color and consistency of any secretions, how the patient tolerated the procedure, and any unusual observations.

PROCEDURE: ASSISTING THE PATIENT WITH LEG EXERCISES

1. Wash your hands.
2. Check the patient's identification bracelet and speak the patient's name.
3. Explain that you are going to help with leg exercises to improve blood flow and prevent blood clots.
4. Follow facility policy for asking visitors to leave the room.
5. Obtain a bath blanket.
6. Close the privacy curtain.
7. Raise the bed to a high level to ease your body movements. Lower the side rail.

8. Place the bath blanket over the patient and fold the top bed linens to the foot of the bed.
9. Position the patient on the back; the head of the bed may be raised for the patient's comfort.
10. For each of the following exercises, help the weak patient as needed. Repeat each exercise 5 times or as instructed.
11. Have the patient rotate the ankles by moving the toes in circles. Repeat with both feet.
12. Have the patient raise the whole leg up from the bed and then back. Repeat, and then repeat with other leg.
13. Support the patient's leg with one hand under the knee and the other under the ankle; have the patient flex the knee by raising the leg up from the bed and bending the knee, then extending it out straight. Repeat, and then repeat with other leg.
14. Have the patient dorsiflex the ankle by bending the foot with toes back toward the leg; then plantarflex the ankle by pointing the toes downward. Repeat, and then repeat with the other foot.
15. Help the patient lie back in bed, and fold the top bed linens back up. Remove the bath blanket.
16. Raise the side rail. Lower the bed to its lowest horizontal position.
17. Make sure the patient is comfortable and can reach the signal light.
18. Open the privacy curtain.
19. Wash your hands.

20. Report to the nurse that you have helped the patient with leg exercises, how the patient tolerated the exercise, and any unusual observations.

Chapter 18
The Elderly Patient

This chapter includes information on the following:
General rules for psychological care
General rules for preventing confusion
General rules to ensure safety

General Rules for Psychological Care

- Because the elderly patient may be undergoing many changes that cause special psychological needs, it is important to provide psychological care while caring for the patient's physical needs.
- Follow the principles for interacting well with patients (see Chapter 1).
- Keep the patient's environment safe, well lit, pleasantly ordered, and as personalized as possible with the patient's things.
- Support and encourage the positive, such as any patient activity and all improvements in the patient's condition, and help minimize anxiety or undue patient concern with the medical condition.
- When talking with the patient, always call the patient by name, speak in nonmedical language, be a good listener, be both friendly and respectful, and touch the patient as appropriate if the patient responds well.
- Try to help the patient maintain a social life with family members, visitors, and other patients and staff.

- When assisting with hygiene, dressing, and personal grooming, help the patient only as needed; do not treat the patient like a child or totally helpless person. Let the patient choose how to dress and make other individual choices.

General Rules for Preventing Confusion

- Help a potentially confused patient stay oriented to reality with gentle reminders of the time of day and date and where the patient is.
- Keep a clock and calendar in the patient's room. Help the patient remember holidays, birthdays, and other special dates and times.
- Always explain who you are and why you are performing any procedure, if the patient seems not to understand; do not assume the patient knows what you are doing simply because you have done it before.
- Help the patient stay in touch with what is happening in the patient's world, whether this means staying in touch with others by telephone or letters or with the outside world through newspapers and television or radio news.
- Speak in simple and clear language and never rush the patient to answer.
- Keep the environment calm and consistent, and care activities routine; have a regular schedule for meals, hygiene, exercise, and so on.
- For a forgetful patient, repeating statements or information is important.

- Do not encourage the patient in any mistaken or forgetful thinking such as thinking someone who has died is still alive.

General Rules to Ensure Safety

- Be sure the patient can always reach the signal light and will not hesitate to use it whenever help is needed.
- Protect the patient by keeping the bed side rails up and the bed in its lowest horizontal position, according to facility policy.
- Remove from the patient's environment any sharp objects, poisonous substances, or potentially dangerous electrical appliances.
- Use a nightlight in the patient's room. Keep a clear path between the bed and the bathroom.
- If the patient tends to wander from the room, monitor the patient--but never restrain a patient just to prevent wandering.
- Encourage the patient who wears glasses or has a hearing aid to use them at all times. Help keep glasses clean.
- Help any patient who is at risk of spilling a hot liquid with a meal or otherwise needs assistance eating. Observe that the patient does not choke on food.
- When getting out of bed, make sure the patient moves slowly, stops to rest sitting on the edge of the bed, and stands with both feet flat on the floor.
- Pay special attention to monitor the patient who smokes.

- Monitor to make sure the patient eats sufficiently and drinks enough water during the day.
- Prevent drafts in the room or sudden temperature changes.
- Prevent the patient from being exposed to infection; discourage visitors with colds or flu from contact with the patient.

Chapter 19
Common Disorders

This chapter includes information on the following:
Principles of care for the cancer patient
Principles of care for the stroke patient
Principles of care for the patient with a heart
problem
Principles of care for the patient with
Alzheimer's
Principles of care for the diabetic patient
Principles of care for the AIDS patient
Principles of care for the hearing impaired
patient
Principles of care for the visually impaired
patient

Principles of Care for the Cancer Patient

► Realizing that many patients may have strong feelings of depression or frustration, be understanding and supportive.

► Because treatments for cancer, such as chemotherapy and radiation, may have many side effects, the patient may need additional care for pain, nausea, vomiting, diarrhea, constipation, and other problems.

► Because some side effects, such as hair loss, or the surgical removal of an organ or body part, such as a breast, can affect the patient's image of self, the patient may need special reassurance and emotional support.

► The cancer patient needs both exercise and sufficient rest.

- ▸ Even though the patient's appetite may be diminished with some treatments, good nutrition and adequate fluid intake are important.
- ▸ Be careful not to avoid the patient or minimize interaction because you're uncomfortable dealing with cancer; often patients just need someone to listen to their feelings.

Principles of Care for the Stroke Patient

- ▸ Because the loss of ability to speak, paralysis, or other loss of function can be devastating psychologically, the patient needs support and encouragement.
- ▸ Much of the care of the stroke patient is rehabilitative, and the patient should be praised and encouraged for even small improvements.
- ▸ Be patient when working with the stroke victim, and encourage the patient not to expect sudden improvements.
- ▸ Help the patient exercise regularly (such as range-of-motion exercises; see Chapter 13 procedure) and encourage coughing and deep breathing (see Chapter 17 procedure).
- ▸ Keep the bed side rails up.
- ▸ If unable to speak, help the patient communicate with other means such as by writing on paper or slate board or using picture cards.
- ▸ If the patient is paralyzed on one side, be alert to help the patient use the strong side in eating, in self-care activities, in getting in or out of a wheelchair, and in other activities.
- ▸ Reposition the patient often and provide care to prevent bedsores (see Chapter 7 procedures).

▸ Assist the patient in gaining as much independence as possible in dressing and grooming, personal hygiene, and other self-care activities.

Principles of Care for the Patient with a Heart Problem

▸ The patient who has had a heart attack is first treated in a coronary care unit, then transferred and started on a rehabilitative program of gradual exercise, dietary and lifestyle changes, and much patient education.
▸ The patient with congestive heart failure may need a special diet, reduced activity, fluid intake and output record, and use of elastic stockings while receiving medical treatment.
▸ The patient with coronary artery disease, such as a partly or fully blocked artery, may experience chest pain (angina) and be treated with medication, rest, reduced activity, diet changes, and education for coping with stress; the goal is to prevent a heart attack or the need for surgery.
▸ It is often important to assure the patient of the need for gradual rehabilitation and to encourage compliance with the doctor's orders for diet, exercise, reduced activity, and self-care.

Principles of Care for the Patient with Alzheimer's

▸ Maintain a consistent, calm, and quiet environment with a daily routine.
▸ Encourage the patient to be active and to engage in interaction and activities with others.

► Help the patient stay oriented to reality (see Chapter 18) and use repetition to help the patient understand and remember key elements of care.

► Follow the principles for caring for the elderly patient: psychological care, preventing confusion, and ensuring safety (see Chapter 18).

► Help family members and visitors accept the patient with Alzheimer's and to cope with changes in the person.

Principles of Care for the Diabetic Patient

► Because urine testing (see Chapter 11 procedures) is important in establishing the patient's dietary and medical treatment needs, be careful to do tests accurately and at the instructed times.

► Help the patient stick to the required diet and avoid foods not allowed.

► Because the diabetic patient is more likely to have circulation problems, help the patient change positions often, avoid crossing the legs, and avoid all nonprescription medicines without the doctor's approval.

► Because the diabetic patient is more likely to have problems with skin breakdown, help the patient remember to always protect the feet by wearing shoes, to avoid all clothing and shoes that are tight or put pressure on the skin, to use warm water rather than hot when bathing and to pat the skin dry carefully, and to tell the nurse or doctor about any changes in how the skin or any body area feels.

- Report to the nurse any observed skin changes or sores, or any patient complaints of numbness, tingling, or other changed sensations.
- Recognize and report to the nurse if you see any of the signs of low blood sugar (also called insulin reaction or hypoglycemia): blurred vision, headache, heavy sweating, dizziness or weakness, nervousness, or disorientation.
- Recognize and report to the nurse if you see any of the signs of high blood sugar (also called diabetic coma or hyperglycemia): dry or flushed skin, lowered or loss of consciousness, heavy breathing, general aches and pains, frequent urination, nausea or vomiting, or a fruity-smelling breath.

Principles of Care for the AIDS Patient

- To protect the patient, other patients, and yourself, always follow the rules for preventing infection (see Chapter 8).
- Use the special precautions for dealing with AIDS patients (see Chapter 8 procedure on page 142).
- Realizing how serious the patient's disease is and the patient's likely strong feelings of depression or frustration, be understanding and supportive.
- Because AIDS is transmitted through body fluids, particularly blood and semen but also possibly through saliva and other fluids, be especially careful when performing procedures involving body fluids.

▸ Since AIDS is not transmitted through casual contact with the patient, do not be fearful of the patient or reluctant to touch the patient in procedures. Such avoidance can be psychologically harmful to the patient.

▸ Many AIDS patients seen in health facilities are dying. Be aware of and help meet the special needs of the dying patient (see Chapter 20).

▸ Because AIDS patients are at high risk for developing other diseases, protect the patient and follow instructions carefully for all procedures for treatment of other conditions.

Principles of Care for the Hearing Impaired Patient

▸ Because hearing loss may be gradual, the patient may not be immediately aware of a hearing impairment. Signs include straining to hear or leaning forward, inattentiveness, asking another to repeat what was said, avoiding conversation, irritation, speaking loudly, or turning the head to use the better ear.

▸ Because the loss of hearing can be very frustrating or depressing, the patient needs support and encouragement.

▸ When communicating with a hearing impaired patient:
   • Minimize other noises, face the patient, and speak clearly and distinctly in a normal tone at normal volume.
   • Let the patient see your face and mouth.
   • If one ear is better, stay on that side of the patient.

- Use simple language and short sentences. Avoid tiring the patient with long conversation.
- When teaching the patient how to do something, carefully show the person the steps of the activity. Do not talk at the same time the patient is looking away from your face to watch the activity.
- Be careful not to startle the patient by approaching closely when you cannot be seen.
- If the patient has a hearing aid, encourage its use and help as needed. Be aware that even with a hearing aid in place, the patient may still have difficulty hearing.

► Help the patient care for a hearing aid:
  - Because the hearing aid is an expensive and delicate instrument, handle it carefully and keep it away from heat, cold, and moisture.
  - Learn how the hearing aid is put on and taken off and help the patient as needed.
  - Learn how to adjust the volume of the hearing aid, asking the patient to tell you when the volume level is comfortable. Learn how to turn it on and off.
  - Encourage the patient to tell you if the hearing aid makes any other sounds or stops working.
  - Make sure a spare battery of the correct size and type is available and that you know how to change the battery.
  - Do not try to clean a hearing aid other than wiping it gently with a tissue.

Principles of Care for the Visually Impaired Patient

- ► Because the loss of vision can be very frustrating or depressing, the patient needs support and encouragement.
- ► A visual impairment may be related to the patient's health problem or may have existed earlier; the patient may be comfortable with the impairment or disturbed and in need of orientation.
- ► Assist a partially sighted patient only to the extent needed. Make sure the patient's room is well lighted and clear of obstructions that could impede movement.
- ► When communicating with a blind patient:
  - Identify yourself before entering the room or approaching closely, and tell the patient when you leave.
  - Always explain, step by step, what you are doing when providing care.
  - Use the patient's sense of touch to show the patient how to use the signal light button, how to find the water glass or tissues, and so on.
  - Help the patient imagine what cannot be seen; for example, explain where items are on the food tray by comparing the tray to a clock face (coffee cup at three o'clock, etc.).
- ► When caring for a blind patient:
  - Help the patient stay oriented to the location of equipment and furniture in the room.

- When walking with the patient, walk slightly ahead, and guide by having the patient hold you arm. Always let the patient know when you are approaching steps, doorways, or other factors that modify the walking.
- Never provide more help than is needed or wanted by the patient; for example, you may help the patient at a meal by opening a container of buttering bread, but do not assume you need to feed the patient.
- Help the patient maintain as much independence as possible in hygiene, grooming, and self-care activities.

Chapter 20
The Dying Patient

This chapter includes information on the following:
The stages of dying
The needs of the dying patient
The signs of approaching death
The signs of death
Procedure: Assisting with postmortem care

The Stages of Dying

► The stages of dying are a pattern of thinking and behaving most patients go through after learning they are dying. Not all patients react the same or move through the stages in the same way or same time.

► In the first stage, called denial, when first informed that the condition or disease will lead to death, the patient may refuse to believe it.

► In the second stage, called anger, the patient feels anger and rage about dying and may blame others.

► In the third stage, called bargaining, the patient is calmer but attempts to bargain with a supreme being or force, making promises if only death will be postponed.

► In the fourth stage, depression, the patient starts to accept dying and now feels grief and may start mourning.

► In the last stage, called acceptance, the patient has accepted the inevitable death and may feel peaceful about it or may withdraw.

The Needs of the Dying Patient

- ► Accept that the dying patient will undergo many stresses and psychological changes after learning that death is coming. Give support to the patient throughout the stages of dying:
  - • The patient in the denial stage may not be able to cope with any care given during this time; be patient and calm, and listen to the patient but do not try to force the patient to accept the coming death.
  - • The patient in anger may lash out at you or others giving care; do not take this personally, but be understanding and accept the patient's anger.
  - • Provide support to the patient during the bargaining stage and understand the patient's inner conflict; do not contradict the patient's attempts to bargain for longer life.
  - • Be a good listener when the patient enters the depression stage, but realize that this stage is normal and do not try to cheer up the patient.
  - • Once the patient accepts dying, provide the best care and support you can but accept the patient's attitude and potential withdrawal from life.
- ► In any stage, the dying patient may have a special need to talk with others and express feelings and concerns; be a good listener.
- ► For a patient who expresses a desire to see a clergyman, rabbi, or other spiritual counselor, cooperate fully to allow others to help the patient with spiritual needs.
- ► Respect the patient's need for privacy alone or with family members or religious counselors.

- Observe the patient's response to your actions and act accordingly; for example, one patient may respond well to being touched, while another may react with anger.
- Family members of the dying patient are also undergoing many psychological changes; be respectful and understanding of their behavior and response to the patient.
- Even if the patient seems unconscious, do not say anything that you would not say otherwise, for the patient may still be able to hear you.
- Be observant of how the patient's physical and personal needs may change as death approaches and the patient becomes more helpless. Be ready to help the patient with care activities that formerly the patient handled independently.
- Pay special attention to the patient's needs for comfort; frequent repositioning may be helpful, the patient may prefer a brightly lit room, and so on.
- A dying patient may need more help in meeting elimination needs (see Chapter 11 procedures) or may require mouth hygiene more frequently (see Chapter 7 procedures).

The Signs of Approaching Death

Note: *Death may come slowly or quickly, depending on the patient and the condition, but the following may be signs of approaching death. Never stop providing care, however, if one or more of these signs is present, as they may be caused by other factors. Report any of these to the nurse.*

► The patient may feel cold regardless of the room temperature and number of blankets on the bed.
► The patient may stop feeling any pain at all and may suddenly seem to become very peaceful.
► Vision may become blurred and gradually fail. Hearing is usually the last sense to be lost.
► Consciousness may give way to stupor or coma, or the patient may be fully conscious until death.
► Blood circulation may slow, making the patient's skin pale and cold to the touch.
► The pulse may become irregular and weak; just before death the pulse may not be felt at all.
► The patient may seem to be staring out at space and not respond to visual stimulus.
► Breathing may become slower, irregular, and more labored. Mucus in the throat and bronchial passages may make the sound called a death rattle. Breathing may stop altogether just before death.
► The muscles may relax completely and the patient's body and face become limp.

The Signs of Death

- The pupils of the eyes are fixed and dilated.
- There are no pulse, respirations, or blood pressure.
- The patient is not considered dead until pronounced dead by the doctor.

PROCEDURE: ASSISTING WITH POSTMORTEM CARE

1. Wash your hands.
2. Check the patient's identification bracelet.
3. Follow facility policy for asking family members or others to leave the room.
4. Collect the following equipment: postmortem care kit (with shroud, bag for personal belongings, identification tags, etc.), towels, wash basin, gown, tape or bandage roll, stretcher, and disposable bed protector.
5. Close the door and privacy curtain.
6. Raise the bed to a high level to ease your body movements. Position the bed flat. Lower the side rail.
7. Position the body on the back, with arms and legs straight and head resting on one pillow.
8. Close the eyelids by gently pulling down on the lashes.
9. Follow facility policy to remove dentures or leave them in the mouth. Close the mouth and if necessary use a rolled towel under the chin to support it closed.
10. Remove all jewelry, following facility policy for whether to leave rings on the hands (secure with tape, if so).

11. Follow instructions to remove tubes, catheters, bandages and dressings.
12. Put the bed protector under any body area to be washed.
13. Carefully wash and dry any soiled areas of the body.
14. Put a clean gown on the body.
15. Put an completed identification tag on the right big toe and on the wrist if facility policy.
16. Put all the patient's belongings in the bag for possessions and label the bag.
17. If the family will be viewing the body, cover it with a clean sheet. Straighten the room and lower the lighting. Give family members a private moment with the deceased patient.
18. When the family has departed, move the body onto the shroud and fold it properly around the body. Use tape or bandage to tie the shroud around the body at the waist, elbows, and knees.
19. Put an identification tag on the shroud.
20. With one or more others, move the body onto the stretcher.
21. Make sure the doors to other patient rooms you will pass are closed.
22. Transport the body to the morgue.
23. Take the bag of jewelry and personal belongings to your facility's appropriate place.
24. Dispose of used supplies and laundry. Strip the bed.
25. Wash your hands.
26. Report to the nurse that you have taken the body to the morgue after giving postmortem care, stripped the bed, and properly stored the bag with belongings.

Chapter 21
Home Health Care

This chapter includes information on the following:
Responsibilities of the home health nursing
assistant
General rules for care in the home
General rules for safety in the home

Responsibilities of the Home Health Nursing Assistant

► Respect the patient's home and all possessions; be careful not to intrude on the privacy of others.
► Follow the principles for interacting with the patient and family members (see Chapter 1).
► You may perform many of the health care procedures described in this book, but never carry out an action you have not been trained or instructed to do for the patient.
► You may transport the patient to appointments with other health care providers.
► You may help with some housekeeping tasks, but generally not heavy cleaning.
► You may prepare meals for the patient; you may also do the grocery shopping.
► You may do laundry for the patient.
► You may help the patient with any of the activities of daily living.
► You may perform other tasks as requested by your supervisor.

General Rules for Care In the Home

- Be prepared for handling any emergency situation. Know what first aid to give for common emergencies (see Chapter 3) and how to quickly call for help.
- Do not try to run the home or change the home patient's cultural or social habits; accept that the patient's lifestyle may be very different from yours.
- Focus your attention on the care of the patient and try to avoid becoming involved in any family problems.
- Housekeeping and other tasks are lower priority than caring for the patient; do not allow these to interfere with care.
- Be flexible in adapting equipment used for procedures in the home; many common home items can be substituted for hospital equipment such as basins, trays, and so on.
- Maintain cleanliness in the house, particularly the bathroom and kitchen, to prevent infection; wash and disinfect equipment appropriately and keep all surfaces clean.
- Keep careful records of all care given to the home patient and all activities performed in the home. Report any unexpected patient changes or unusual observations at any time to your supervisor.

General Rules for Safety in the Home

- Post near the telephone the numbers for the doctor, hospital, ambulance, supervising nurse, poison control center, and fire and police departments.
- If the home patient seems to be experiencing a medical emergency, do not delay care by trying to reach your supervisor or the doctor--call for emergency assistance immediately.
- Follow all rules for fire, electrical, and patient safety as in a facility (see Chapter 2 rules on pages 11-13).
- Know how best to move the patient out of the house from any room; if the patient is helpless, be prepared to use an emergency drag or carry if necessary.
- Prevent fires from occurring:
  - Monitor carefully a patient who smokes.
  - Do not leave matches where the patient or a child may find them.
  - Make sure clothing, furniture, and other objects are kept away from space heaters, fireplaces, and other dangerously hot areas.
  - Always check the condition of appliance electrical cords and extension cords before using the appliance.
  - Be sure the home is equipped with smoke detectors in the appropriate places and a fire extinguisher at least in the kitchen.
  - If possible, avoid using flammable liquids such as cleaning fluids; if necessary, use with care and do not leave wet objects or areas unattended.

- Watch for safety hazards throughout the home
  and prevent accidents from occurring:
  - Medications or liquids that may cause
    poisoning
  - Dangerous or sharp equipment
  - Electrical appliances or wiring that may be
    faulty
  - Loose rugs that may slip underfoot
  - Flammable liquid or cleaning equipment
  - Wet floor areas that may cause a slip
  - Objects on floor that may cause a trip and
    fall

Appendix A
Medical Abbreviations

abd	abdomen
ac or a.c.	before meals
ad lib	as desired
ADL	activities of daily living
A.M. or a.m. or am	morning
amb	ambulatory
amt	amount
approx	approximately
b.i.d. or bid	twice a day
BM or b.m.	bowel movement
BP	blood pressure
B.R. or BR	bed rest
BRP or B.R.P.	bathroom privileges
BSC	bedside commode
C	centigrade or celsius
Ca	cancer
Cath	catheter
CBC	complete blood count (lab test)
CBR or C.B.R.	complete bed rest
cc	cubic centimeter
CCU	coronary care unit
CPR	cardiopulmonary resuscitation
CVA	cerebrovascular accident
dc or d/c	discontinue
DOA	dead on arrival
drsg	dressing
DX or Dx	diagnosis
ECG or EKG	electrocardiogram
EEG	electroencephalogram

ER	emergency room
F	Fahrenheit
FBS	fasting blood sugar (lab test)
FF or F.F.	forced fluids
ft	foot
Fx urine	fresh fractional urine
gal	gallon
GI	gastrointestinal
Gyn	gynecology
H_2O	water
hr	hour
HS or hs	hour of sleep
ht	height
HWB	hot water bottle
ICU	intensive care unit
in	inch
I&O	intake and output
isol	isolation
IV	intravenous
L	liter
lab	laboratory
lb	pound
liq	liquid
LPN	licensed practical nurse
LVN	licensed vocational nurse
MD	medical doctor
med	medication
min	minute
ml	milliliter
mn or m/n or mid noc	midnight
NA or N/A	nurse assistant
NG	nasogastric
noc or noct	at night
NPO	nothing by mouth

O_2	oxygen
OB	obstetrics
OJ	orange juice
OOB	out of bed
OR	operating room
ord	orderly
OT	occupational therapy
oz	ounce
PAR or **P.A.R.**	postanaesthesia room
pc or **p.c.**	after meals
Peds	pediatrics
P.M. or **p.m.** or **pm**	after noon
p.o. or **po**	by mouth
postop	postoperative
preop	preoperative
prep	preparation (skin prep)
prn or **p.r.n.**	whenever needed
pt	patient
PT	physical therapy
q	every
q.a.m. or **qam**	every morning
q.d. or **qd**	every day
q.h. or **qh**	every hour
q2h q3h q4h	every 2 hours, every 3 hours, every 4 hours
q.h.s. or **qhs**	every night at bedtime
q.i.d. or **qid**	four times every day
q.o.d. or **qod**	every other day
qt	quart
R or **r**	rectal (temperature)
RN	registered nurse
ROM or **rom**	range of motion
RR	recovery room
s	without
sol	solution

spec	specimen
SSE	soap suds enema
STD	sexually transmitted disease
stat	immediately
surg	surgery
tbsp	tablespoon
t.i.d. or **tid**	three times a day
TLC	tender loving care
TPR	temperature, pulse, and respirations
tsp	teaspoon
U/A or **u/a**	urinalysis
VD	venereal disease
VSE or **V.S.**	vital signs
WBC	white blood count (lab test)
w/c	wheelchair
wt	weight

Appendix B
Glossary

A

Abdomen - the part of the body in front above the pelvis and below the chest

Abduct - to move the arm or leg out away from the body; compare to adduct

Absorb - the action by which one thing soaks up or takes in another

Accountability - legal and ethical responsibility to give the best possible care

Acetest - a commercially prepared urine test

Acquired immune deficiency syndrome (AIDS) - a fatal communicable disease transmitted through body fluids

Active range-of-motion (ROM) exercises - exercises in which the patient moves the joints through their full range of movements; compare to passive ROM exercises

Activities of daily living - all the activities the patient or any person carries out daily, such as eating, dressing, and personal hygiene

Acute illness - an illness or condition that develops suddenly and may become serious quickly; compare to chronic illness

Adduct - to move the arm or leg in toward the body; compare to abduct

Admit - the formal process by which the person becomes a patient within the health care facility

AIDS - see acquired immune deficiency syndrome

Airway - the route through which air reaches the lungs and which may be obstructed in a breathing emergency: includes the mouth, pharynx, trachea, and bronchial tubes

Alveoli - air sacs in the lungs where oxygen enters the blood

Alzheimer's disease - common nervous system disease of the elderly in which the patient gradually loses mental functioning

Ambulation - walking

Ambulatory - a patient who can walk independently

Anal - referring to the area around the anus

Anatomy - the study of body structures; compare to physiology

Anesthesia - the state in which feeling is lost in one local area of the body or generally throughout

Anesthetic - a drug that leads to anesthesia, such as used for surgery

Angina - a type of severe chest pain caused by certain heart conditions

Ankle restraint - made of a bandage or other material restricting the movement of the patient's ankle, used to limit the patient's movements

Anterior - referring to the front of the body or body part; compare to posterior

Anus - the opening from the rectum to the outside, through which bowel movements occur

Aphasia - loss of the ability to speak or understand language, such as may occur after a stroke

Apical pulse - the pulse as felt over the heart

Artery - a blood vessel that moves blood from the heart to the body; compare to vein

Asepsis - a state in which microorganisms are not present, such as with sterile instruments or after disinfection

Aspirate - to suck in a substance, such as to aspirate fluid from a body area with a needle or to accidentally breathe in a liquid

Assessment - an evaluation of the patient's condition

Atrophy - a state in which muscles waste away when not used

Axillary - referring to the armpits

B

Bacteria - a type of microorganism that may cause disease; can be killed with a disinfectant

Bargaining - a psychological stage in which the dying person attempts to live longer by making promises of some changed behavior

Bedpan - a pan used by bedridden patients for urinary or bowel elimination

Bedridden - a patient whose condition does not allow movement from bed

Bedsore - see decubitus ulcer

Benign - a growth or tumor that does not spread or grow back if surgically removed; compare to malignant

Binder - a type of cloth bandage, usually wide, used to hold something in place

Bladder - sac-like organ in the abdomen that holds urine until it is urinated

Blood pressure (BP) - a measure of how forcefully the blood is flowing through an artery or vein

Body alignment - the straight line position of the body, such as lying with back and neck straight, arms straight at sides, and legs straight and extended fully
Body language - expressions, gestures, and body movements that can communicate a feeling or thought to another person
Body mechanics - principles of moving the body in a safe and efficient manner
Bowel elimination - the process of passing feces out through the anus; also called defecation
Bronchial - referring to the lower part of the airway where air is brought into the lungs

C
Calibration - markings on a container for measurement
Calories (cal) - measurement of energy in foods
Cancer - any of many types of serious and malignant growths or tumors
Carbohydrates - a basic food substance, including sugar and starch
Cardiac arrest - condition in which the heart stops
Cardiopulmonary resuscitation (CPR) - emergency procedure to keep alive a person whose heart and breathing have stopped
Cast - a casing, made of plaster or another hard substance, to protect and immobilize a limb or body part with a fractured bone
Catheter - a tube for draining out a liquid, such as urine from the bladder
Celsius (C) - a temperature scale where water freezes at 0 degrees and boils at 100 degrees; compare to Fahrenheit
Centigrade (C) - another term for celsius scale

Central nervous system (CNS) - body system consisting of the brain, spinal cord, and nerves, which regulates all body functions

Cerebral - referring to a part of the brain

Cerebrospinal fluid - a fluid around the brain and spinal cord

Cerebrovascular accident (CVA) - a condition in which a part of the brain is damaged by not receiving enough blood; also called a stroke

Chart - the patient's medical record

Chronic illness - a usually incurable illness or condition that develops slowly and may last a long time; compare to acute illness

Circulation - the movement of blood throughout the body

Circulatory system - the body system consisting of the heart, arteries, and veins and other organs that make and help move the blood

Circumcised - the state in which a section of the foreskin of the penis has been removed at birth, often done routinely

Clean catch urine - urine collected for a specimen, with the sample taken after the flow or urine starts, in order to minimize contamination

Cleansing enema - enema given to promote emptying the lower bowel of feces and to clean the bowel and rectum

Clinitest - a commercially prepared urine test

Closed bed - a made-up bed that is not currently being used by a patient; compare to open bed

Colostomy - an opening made between the colon and the outside of the abdomen to allow passage of feces

Coma - a state of unconsciousness caused by illness or medical condition

Commode - a chair-like device with a bedpan that can be moved to the bedside

Communicable disease - a disease one person can catch from another; also called contagious or infectious

Complication - a health problem that may result from the patient's condition or some aspect of treatment

Compress - a pad or cloth used to apply warmth or cold to an area of the skin

Congestive heart failure (CHF) - an illness in which the heart does not pump effectively

Constipation - the condition in which the patient does not defecate regularly or recently

Contaminated - the state in which an instrument, surface, or any object is considered not free of microorganisms

Contracture - a muscle condition in which the muscle stays contracted rather than stretching back out after contracting

Convalescence - the period when the patient is recuperating after an operation or illness

Convulsion - strong muscular contractions as in a seizure

Cyanotic - referring to skin or membranes that turns bluish when the patient's blood is not carrying enough oxygen

Cubic centimeter (cc) - standard unit of measure for liquids

D

Decubitus ulcer - a skin sore or condition usually caused by pressure on an area when the patient is immobile for long periods; also called bedsore or pressure sore

Defecate - to have a bowel movement
Dehydration - a state in which the body is lacking enough fluid for full normal functioning
Denial - the first stage of dying in which the person does not accept the truth about dying
Depression - a psychological state of sadness; also a stage of dying before the person accepts the coming death
Diabetes - a metabolic disorder that can be treated but not completely cured
Diagnosis - the determination of the exact nature of a patient's illness or disease
Diarrhea - a condition in which the person has unusually frequent and watery bowel movements
Diastolic blood pressure - the blood pressure when the heart is in the resting state between beats; compare to systolic blood pressure
Digestion - the process in which the digestive system breaks down food into nutrients
Dilated - the state of being larger, such as dilated pupils of the eyes
Disability - the state of not being able to function fully or normally
Discharge - the formal process of checking a patient out of the health care facility
Disinfect - to kill microorganisms on a surface, instrument, or other object with a disinfecting solution, a process of heat, or other method
Disoriented - psychological state of being confused, unable to remember obvious things, or not grasping reality
Disposable - referring to equipment or supplies designed to be used only once and then discarded
Distended - swollen

Dorsiflex - to move a joint so that the body part such as the foot moves backward; compare to plantarflex

Double-voided urine specimen - a fresh urine specimen collected 30 minutes after the patient has urinated stale urine; also called a fresh-fractional urine specimen

Douche - a cleansing flow of water, such as vaginal irrigation

Drape - a covering for the patient's body during a procedure

Drawsheet - a small sheet used on the middle of the bottom sheet to help protect the bottom linens and to help move a patient

E

Edema - a swollen area of the body such as the legs or ankles caused by fluid collecting

Eggcrate mattress - a pad made of foam shaped like an eggcrate used to prevent decubitus ulcers

Elastic bandage - a stretchy wide bandage wrapped around an area of a limb to improve circulation

Elastic stockings - special stretchy stockings applied to the feet and legs to improve circulation

Elbow restraint - made of a bandage or other material restricting the movement of the patient's elbow, used to limit the patient's movements

Elimination - the process of removing urine or feces from the body; urination or bowel movement

Embolus - a blood clot that lodges in a small blood vessel

Emergency - a patient's life-threatening condition requiring immediate action or first aid

Emesis - another word for vomitus

Emesis basin - basin designed to collect fluid, saliva, or vomit from the patient's mouth

Empathy - the ability to understand and feel what the patient is feeling without making judgments

Enema - the process of bringing fluid through a tube into the rectum for cleansing or other purposes

Epidermis - the outer layer of the skin

Esophagus - the tube that carries food from the throat to the stomach

Ethical - referring to acting responsibly and according to commonly accepted practices

Evacuation - a term sometimes used for defecation or bowel movement

Excretion - same as elimination

Exhale - to breathe air and carbon dioxide out from the lungs

Expectorate - to cough up sputum or other material from the lungs or airway

Extend - to move a joint such that the body part is moved straight out; compare to flex

F

Face mask - a device covering the nose and mouth to give the patient oxygen

Fahrenheit (F) - a temperature scale where water freezes at 32 degrees and boils at 212 degrees; compare to Celsius

Fan-fold - a way to fold the top bed linen to the foot of the bed

Feces - the solid waste matter eliminated in a bowel movement; also called stool

Fever - condition in which the person's temperature is above the normal 98.6 degrees F

First aid - the initial care given to a person with a health problem or in an emergency

Flatus - gas that develops in the intestines and is eliminated through the anus

Flex - to move a joint such that the body part is bent, such as the elbow or knee; compare to extend

Fluid balance - a normal body condition in which as much fluid is eliminated from the body as is taken in

Fluid intake - the total fluid taken into the body through all routes, such as ingesting it or receiving fluid by intravenous needle

Fluid output - the total fluid eliminated from the body through all routes, including urination, defecation, sweating, and other mechanisms

Flushed - referring to a red skin appearance

Foot drop - condition in which the foot is in plantarflexion

Forced fluids - a doctor's order for the patient to be given more than usual amounts of fluids

Foreskin - loose skin at the tip of the penis

Fracture - a broken bone

Fresh urine - urine that has not been in long in the bladder; see double-voided urine specimen

G

Gait belt - another term for transfer belt

Gastrointestinal (GI) system - the body system consisting of the stomach, intestines, and other organs for the digestion of food

Gavage - the process of feeding a patient through a nasogastric tube

General - Referring to the whole body; compare to localized

General anesthetic - a drug that leads to general anesthesia for the whole body, such as used for surgery

Geriatric - referring to an elderly patient

Glucose - a kind of sugar

Graduate - a container with calibrated markings for measuring fluids

Gurney - see stretcher

H

Hazard - any condition in the environment that is unsafe or could cause an accident

Head nurse - a supervisor of nurses and nurse assistants

Hearing impaired - a patient who is deaf or has less than normal hearing function

Heart attack - a condition in which the blood supply to heart tissue is interrupted; also called myocardial infarction

Heat lamp - a special kind of lamp used to apply heat to an area of the patient's body

Heat pad - a device, usually electrical, for direct application of heat to a patient's skin

Hemorrhage - bleeding

Hormone - a body substance produced for a specific and necessary effect in an organ or body system

Hospice - a program or place for dying patients; may be in the home

Hygiene - the daily routines and procedures for preserving body cleanliness and sanitary conditions

Hyperextend - to extend a joint beyond its normal straight position; compare to extend

Hyperglycemia - diabetic condition in which there is too much sugar in the blood

Hypertension - the condition of having abnormally high blood pressure

Hyperventilation - breathing that is faster than normal; may be deeper or more shallow than normal

Hypoglycemia - diabetic condition in which there is too little sugar in the blood

I

Immobile - confined to bed or otherwise unable to move

Impacted - referring to hard stool that cannot leave the rectum normally

Incident - any unusual thing that happens in the facility that should be reported

Incontinent - referring to a patient who lacks control over urination or defecation

Indwelling catheter - a urinary drainage tube that is left in position

Infection - a condition in which microorganisms have entered the body to cause disease

Inflammation - a condition of body tissues responding to illness or a condition, causing redness and swelling

Inhale - to breathe air and oxygen into the lungs

Insulin - a hormone needed for metabolism and not produced in normal amounts in diabetics

Insulin shock - condition in a diabetic caused by too much insulin

Intake and output - system for measuring and recording a patient's fluid intake and output; see fluid intake, fluid output

Integumentary system - the body system consisting of the skin, hair, and nails

Intermittent - starting and stopping, not continuous, such as intermittent traction

Intravenous (IV) - referring to injection into a vein, such as giving IV fluids

Invasion of privacy - an unethical and illegal act of sharing private information about a person without the person's consent

Isolation - condition of keeping a patient protected from the possibility of infection, or keeping others from being infected by the patient; a special room and special techniques for gowns and masks may be sued

J

Jacket restraint - a special jacket-like restraint to keep the patient from falling out of bed or a wheelchair

Joint - the area where two bones are joined together with tendons and muscles

K

Ketostix - a commercially prepared urine test

Kilogram (kg) - basic unit of weight in the metric system, the equivalent of about 2.2 pounds

L

Lateral - referring to the side, such as lying on one's side in a lateral position

Liability - Legal responsibility for one's actions and for giving the best possible care by current standards

Licensed practical nurse (LPN) - a type of nurse usually with one year of education, compared to the two or more years of training for registered nurses (RN)

Licensed vocational nurse (LVN) - another term for an LPN

Lift - special device for lifting and moving the patient, such as from bed to a wheelchair

Local anesthetic - a drug that leads to anesthesia in one specific area of the body, such as used for surgery

Localized - Referring to a specific part of the body; compare to general

Lubricant - creamy substance such as petroleum jelly to reduce friction between two surfaces

M

Malignant - a serious growth or tumor that may spread or grow back if surgically removed; compare to benign

Malpractice - legal term for acting negligently, not giving the best possible care in accordance with current standards; grounds for a lawsuit

Medical asepsis - asepsis for routine medical purposes in the health facility; see asepsis; compare to surgical asepsis

Membrane - a thin tissue layer, usually over another tissue

Menstruation - a woman's monthly period of uterine blood loss

Metabolism - the processes by which body cells take in and give out substances, including nutrients, oxygen, and fluid

Metastasis - spreading of cancer cells from one tissue to another

Microorganism - a microscopic organism that may cause disease, including bacteria, viruses, and fungi

Micturate - another term for urinate

Midstream urine specimen - urine specimen collected midway through the urination

Mitered - referring to the folding of sheets when making a hospital bed

Mitt restraint - a restraint like a mitten that fits over the patient's hand to restrict the movement of the hand

Mobile - able to move about, not bedridden

Mucus - a substance secreted in the nose, lungs, and other areas

Muscular system - the body system of muscles, tendons, and ligaments primarily for supporting and moving the body

Myocardial infarction - see heart attack

N

Nasal cannula - device for delivering oxygen through the nostrils

Nasogastric tube - tube that runs through one nostril and to the stomach, for feeding or other medical purposes

Negligence - not giving the best possible care according to current standards; grounds for a lawsuit

Neoplasm - a cancerous growth

Nervous system - see central nervous system

Nonambulatory - referring to a patient not able to walk independently

Nosocomial infection - an infection the patient gets while in the hospital

Nothing by mouth (NPO) - doctor's order for the patient to receive no food or fluid, such as before surgery

Nurse assistant - person trained to help the nurse provide care for the patient

Nursing care plan - a written method for planning and giving nursing care

O

Observation - the act of observing and monitoring the patient for any change in condition

Obstetrical - referring to health care related to pregnancy and childbirth

Obstruction - a blockage, such as an obstructed airway

Occupational therapist - health professional trained to help the patient function independently in life

Oil retention enema - a type of enema given to soften impacted feces; see enema, see impaction

Open bed - a made-up bed being used by a patient, with the top linen folded down

Oral hygiene - procedures to maintain cleanliness of the mouth

Order - an instruction from the doctor or nurse supervisor for some aspect of patient care

Orthopedic - referring to health care related to bones, joints, and muscles

Ostomy - a surgically made opening from some part of the patient's intestines to the outside of the abdomen for the passing of feces

Ostomy appliance - a device to collect feces through the ostomy site

Oxygen therapy - any of various methods of giving the patient oxygen, such as through a nasal cannula, face mask, or oxygen tent

P

Pallor - pale appearance of the skin

Paralyzed - condition in which the patient cannot move one or more parts of the body

Parenteral - referring to an intravenous process, such as the parental giving of fluids; see intravenous

Passive range-of-motion (ROM) exercises - exercises in which the nurse or other moves the patient's joints through their full range of movements; compare to active range-of-motion exercises

Pathogen - a microorganism that can cause disease

Patient unit - the patient's room or section of a room and the equipment in it

Pediatric - referring to health care given to children

Perineal area - the area between the thighs from the genitals to the anus

Physical therapist (PT) - health professional trained to help the patient regain abilities to move

Physician - doctor; any of many medically trained specialists

Physiological - referring to something physical, rather than psychological

Physiology - the study of body functioning; compare to anatomy

Plantarflex - to move a joint so that the body part such as the foot moves forward; compare to dorsiflex

Poison - any substance that impedes normal functions when taken into the body; also called toxin

Posterior - referring to the back of the body or body part; compare to anterior

Postmortem - after death

Postoperative (postop) - after surgery

Postpartum - after giving birth

Preoperative (preop) - before surgery

Pressure sore - see decubitus ulcer

Primary nursing - a system of organizing health care in which registered nurses are responsible for the primary patient care

Pronate - to move a joint so that the body part moves outward, such as turning the bottom of the foot outward; compare to supinate

Prone - in the position lying face down

Prosthesis - an artificial body part, such as an artificial eye or leg

Psychological - referring to the mind, feelings, and thoughts; compare to physiological

Pulmonary - referring to the lungs

Pulse - the force one can feel in the arteries caused by the heartbeat; the measurement of number of heartbeats per minute

Pulse deficit - a problem when the radial pulse does not equal the number of heartbeats per minute felt over the heart

R

Radial pulse - the pulse taken at the wrist artery

Range of motion (ROM) exercises - exercises in which the patient or other moves the patient's joints through their full range of movements; compare active and passive ROM

Rectal - referring to the rectum

Rectal irrigation - procedure for cleansing the rectum with a stream of water

Rectal tube - a tube inserted into the rectum from the outside to relieve intestinal gas

Rectum - the lowest section of the large intestine, immediately inside the anus

Registered nurse (RN) - a type of nurse usually with two or more years of education, compared to the one year of training for a licensed practical nurse (LPN)

Rehabilitation - the system of procedures and care to help the patient regain functioning after an illness or condition

Reproductive system - the body system consisting of the male and female reproductive organs

Respiratory system - the body system consisting of the lungs, airway, and other organs for breathing

Restraint - a device to protect the patient from potential harm caused by moving a specific body area or the whole body

Retention - the holding in of something

Rhythm - the regularity or irregularity of the heartbeat or breathing

Rotate - to move a joint such that the body part moves around its center

Rupture - to burst or start leaking

S

Safety belt - a type of restraint that wraps around the patient's waist and is secured and prevents falling out of bed or a wheelchair

Scrotum - the sac-like area beneath the penis, containing the testes

Secretion - to produce and give out a substance, such as glands secreting hormones

Seizure - an epileptic attack or convulsion

Self-care - health and hygiene activities the patient is able to do independently

Shallow breathing - breathing in which the lungs do not fully expand

Shock - a serious condition when an adequate blood supply does not reach the body

Sign - objective information about a patient's condition, such as vital signs, which can be observed and measured; compare to symptom

Sitz bath - a warm bath in which the patient's buttocks and hips are immersed

Skeletal system - the body system consisting of the bones

Skin preparation (prep) - the procedure of washing and shaving a part of the body in preparation for surgery

Solution - a liquid in which another substance is dissolved, such as a soap solution for an enema

Spasm - a sudden muscular contraction

Specimen - a sample taken for laboratory tests, such as a urine or sputum sample

Sphygmomanometer - device for measuring blood pressure

Splint - device used to immobilize a body part

Sputum - mucus and other material that can be coughed up from the lungs

Stages of dying - psychological phases a patient undergoes when learning he or she is dying

Sterilize - to kill all microorganisms on an instrument or surface